W9-BKD-105

The Basic Food & Brand-Name Carbohydrate Counter (*Excerpted from* "*The Dictionary of Calories and Carbohydrates*")

BARBARA KRAUS

Grosset & Dunlap
Publishers, New York

Copyright © 1971, 1973, 1974 by Barbara Kraus

All rights reserved

Published simultaneously in Canada

ISBN: 0-448-11685-5

1976 PRINTING

Printed in the United States of America

(*Excerpted from* The Dictionary of Calories and Carbohydrates)

For Mon Ling, Karl and Ling Ling Landegger

INTRODUCTION

Most of the data presented here are derived from my book THE DICTIONARY OF CALORIES AND CARBOHYDRATES. In that book, 9,000 brand names and basic foods were listed with their calories and carbohydrate count.

In this smaller book I have made certain compromises: whereas in the giant book there were several physical descriptions, here there is but one; when there is only one carbohydrate variation between products the products have been grouped together. Such variations are unimportant and often are only the result of a different way of rounding numbers. Finally, no dietetic products are included that are dietetic only because they are sodium restricted because the carbohydrates are not affected.

For you who have never before had an interest in weight control, I offer the following necessary information.

Carbohydrates

Carbohydrates — which include sugars, starches, and acids — are one of several chemical compounds in food that yield calories. Proteins, found mainly in beef, poultry and fish; fats, found in oils, butter, marbling of meat, poultry skin; and alcohol, found in some beverages, also contribute calories. Except for the alcohol, most foods contain at least some of all these nutrients.

The amount of carbohydrates varies from zero in meats and a trace in alcohol to a heavy concentration in sugar, syrups, some fruits, grains and root vegetables.

As of this date, the most respected nutritional researchers insist that some carbohydrate is necessary every day for maintaining good health. The amount to be included is an individual matter and any drastic effort to change your eating patterns, should be checked with your doctor first.

ABBREVIATIONS AND SYMBOLS

* = prepared as packaging directs[1]
< = less than
& = and
" = inch
canned − bottles or jars as well as cans
dia. = diameter
fl. = fluid
liq. = liquid
lb. = pound
med. = medium

oz. = ounce
pkg. = package
pt. = pint
qt. = quart
sq. = square
T. = tablespoon
Tr. = trace
tsp. = teaspoon
wt. = weight

Italics or name in parentheses = registered trademark, ®.
All data not identified by company or trademark are based upon material obtained from the United States Department of Agriculture.

EQUIVALENTS

By Weight

1 pound = 16 ounces
1 ounce = 28.35 grams
3.52 ounces = 100 grams

By Volume

1 quart = 4 cups
1 cup = 8 fluid ounces
1 cup = ½ pint
1 cup = 16 tablespoons
2 tablespoons = 1 fluid ounce
1 tablespoon = 3 teaspoons
1 pound butter = 4 sticks or 2 cups

[1]If the package directions call for whole or skim milk, the data given here are for whole milk, unless otherwise stated.

Food and Description	Measure or Quantity	Carbohydrates (grams)

A

ABALONE:
Raw, meat only	4 oz.	3.9
Canned	4 oz.	2.6

AC'CENT | ¼ tsp. | 0.

ALMOND:
In shell	4 oz.	11.3
Shelled, whole	1 oz.	5.5
Blanched, slivered (Blue Diamond)	1 cup	33.9
Flavored (Blue Diamond)	1 oz.	9.5
Roasted, diced (Blue Diamond)	1 oz.	5.5

ALPHA-BITS (Post) | 1 oz. | 23.0

AMBROSIA, chilled (Kraft) | 4 oz. | 14.7

ANCHOVY PASTE (Crosse & Blackwell) | 1 oz. | 2.0

ANCHOVY, PICKLED | 1 oz. | <.1

ANGEL FOOD CAKE MIX:
*(Betty Crocker):
1 step	1 cake	314.4
2 step	1 cake	273.6
Confetti	1 cake	321.6
Lemon custard	1 cake	312.0
Strawberry	1 cake	325.2
*(Duncan Hines)	1 cake	355.2
(Pillsbury) raspberry swirl	1 oz.	23.6
(Pillsbury) white	1 oz.	23.3
*(Swans Down)	1 cake	356.4

APPLE:
Eaten with skin	1 lb.	60.5
Eaten without skin	1 lb.	55.0
Dehydrated, uncooked	1 oz.	26.1
Dried, uncooked (Del Monte)	1 cup	54.6
Frozen, sweetened, slices	4 oz.	27.6

*Prepared as Package Directs

Food and Description	Measure or Quantity	Carbohydrates (grams)
APPLE BUTTER:		
(Bama)	1 T.	7.6
(Smucker's)	1 T.	7.6
APPLE CIDER, cherry or sweet		
(Mott's)	½ cup	14.6
APPLE DRINK:		
(Del Monte)	6 fl. oz.	23.6
(Hi-C)	6 fl. oz	22.2
APPLE JACKS (Kellogg's)	1 oz.	25.8
APPLE JELLY:		
(White House)	1 T.	13.0
Low calorie (Slenderella)	1 T.	6.4
APPLE JUICE (Heinz)	5½-fl.-oz. can	21.7
APPLE PIE:		
(Drake's)	2-oz. pie	25.2
(Tastykake)	4-oz. pie	58.6
Frozen:		
(Banquet)	5-oz. serving	49.5
(Morton)	20-oz. pie	202.2
(Morton)	24-oz. pie	240.6
(Morton)	46-oz. pie	459.2
(Mrs. Smith's)	8″ pie	240.0
(Mrs. Smith's) natural juice	9″ pie	390.0
(Mrs. Smith's)	10″ pie	420.0
Dutch apple (Mrs. Smith's)	8″ pie	270.0
Tart (Mrs. Smith's)	8″ pie	250.0
APPLE PIE FILLING:		
(Comstock)	½ cup	45.6
French (Comstock)	½ cup	41.7
(Lucky Leaf)	8 oz.	60.8
Unsweetened (Lucky Leaf)	8 oz.	23.2
APPLESAUCE:		
Sweetened:		
(Del Monte)	½ cup	32.5
(Hunt's)	5-oz. can	25.2

*Prepared as Package Directs

Food and Description	Measure or Quantity	Carbohydrates (grams)
(Seneca) cinnamon	½ cup	30.2
(Seneca) 100% McIntosh	½ cup	30.2
(Stokely-Van Camp)	½ cup	28.5
(White House)	½ cup	28.2
Unsweetened:		
(Blue Boy)	4 oz.	10.4
(Diet Delight)	½ cup	14.2
(Mott's)	½ cup	13.4
(S and W) *Nutradiet*, low calorie	4 oz.	13.7
(S and W) *Nutradiet*, unsweetened	4 oz.	13.6
(Tillie Lewis)	½ cup	12.2
(White House)	½ cup	12.2
APPLESAUCE CAKE MIX, raisin (Duncan Hines)	1 cake	39.0
APPLE TURNOVER (Pepperidge Farm)	3.3-oz. turnover	30.2
APRICOT:		
Fresh, whole	1 lb.	54.6
Canned, regular pack:		
(Del Monte)	½ cup	27.4
(Hunt's)	½ cup	26.9
(Stokely-Van Camp)	½ cup	26.0
Canned, low calorie:		
(Diet Delight)	½ cup	14.9
(S and W) *Nutradiet*, low calorie, whole	2 whole	7.2
(S and W) *Nutradiet*, low calorie, halves	4 halves	9.6
(S and W) *Nutradiet*, unsweetened, halves	4 halves	9.1
(Tillie Lewis)	½ cup	11.2
Dehydrated, uncooked	4 oz.	95.9
Dried, uncooked (Del Monte)	½ cup	39.2
APRICOT LIQUEUR (Leroux) 60 proof	1 fl. oz.	8.9
APRICOT NECTAR (Heinz)	5½-fl.-oz. can	21.0

*Prepared as Package Directs

Food and Description	Measure or Quantity	Carbohydrates (grams)
APRICOT PIE FILLING:		
(Comstock)	1 cup	78.5
(Lucky Leaf)	8 oz.	77.6
APRICOT & PINEAPPLE NECTAR		
(S and W) *Nutradiet*	4 oz.	8.5
APRICOT & PINEAPPLE PRESERVE:		
Sweetened (Bama)	1 T.	13.5
Low calorie (Diet Delight)	1 T.	5.1
AQUAVIT (Leroux) 90 proof	1 fl. oz.	Tr.
ARTICHOKE, Globe or French:		
Raw	1 lb.	19.2
Frozen, hearts (Birds Eye)	5-6 hearts	4.8
ASPARAGUS:		
Raw	1 lb.	12.7
Canned:		
Cut spears & liq. (Green Giant)	10½-oz. can	6.0
Spears & liq. (Green Giant)	15-oz. can	8.4
Frozen:		
Cuts (Birds Eye)	10-oz. pkg.	9.9
Cut spears in butter sauce (Green Giant)	9-oz. pkg.	12.0
Spears (Birds Eye)	10-oz. pkg.	10.8
Spears with Hollandaise sauce (Birds Eye)	10-oz. pkg.	9.6
AUNT JEMIMA SYRUP	8 fl. oz.	216.0
AVOCADO, whole	1 lb.	21.4
*AWAKE (Birds Eye)	½ cup	12.6
AYDS	1 piece	4.9

B

BABY FOOD:		
Apple:		
& apricot, junior (Beech-Nut)	7¾ oz.	51.2
& apricot, strained (Beech-Nut)	4¾ oz.	29.7

*Prepared as Package Directs

Food and Description	Measure or Quantity	Carbohydrates (grams)
& cranberry, junior (Heinz)	7¾ oz.	46.6
& cranberry, strained (Heinz)	4¾ oz.	30.7
& honey, junior (Heinz)	7½ oz.	36.9
& honey with tapioca, strained (Heinz)	4½ oz.	21.8
& pear, junior (Heinz)	7¾ oz.	43.7
& pear, strained (IIeinz)	4½ oz.	26.4
Dutch, dessert (Gerber):		
Junior	7⁸/₁₀ oz.	47.8
Strained	4⁷/₁₀ oz.	28.5
Apple-apricot juice, strained (Heinz)	4½ fl. oz.	22.4
Apple Betty (Beech-Nut):		
Junior	7¾ oz.	55.2
Strained	4¾ oz.	34.8
Apple-cherry juice:		
Strained (Beech-Nut)	4¹/₅ fl. oz. (4.4 oz.)	18.4
Strained (Gerber)	4¹/₅ fl. oz. (4.6 oz.)	14.2
Strained (Heinz)	4½ fl. oz.	21.1
Apple-grape juice:		
Strained (Beech-Nut)	4¹/₅ fl. oz. (4.4 oz.)	20.1
Strained (Heinz)	4½ fl. oz.	22.3
Apple juice:		
Strained (Beech-Nut)	4¹/₅ fl. oz. (4.4 oz.)	14.4
Strained (Gerber)	4¹/₅ fl. oz. (4.6 oz.)	16.0
Strained (Heinz)	4½ fl. oz.	21.7
Apple pie (Heinz):		
Junior	7¾ oz.	49.5
Strained	4¾ oz.	30.0
Apple-pineapple juice, strained (Heinz)	4½ fl. oz.	22.5
Apple-prune & honey (Heinz):		
Junior	7½ oz.	43.8
With tapioca, strained	4½ oz.	25.4
Apple-prune juice, strained (Heinz)	4½ fl. oz.	22.0
Applesauce:		
Junior (Beech-Nut)	7¾ oz.	47.7
Junior (Gerber)	7⁸/₁₀ oz.	44.6
Junior (Heinz)	7¾ oz.	44.7
Strained (Beech-Nut)	4¾ oz.	29.5
Strained (Gerber)	4⁷/₁₀ oz.	27.4

*Prepared as Package Directs

Food and Description	Measure or Quantity	Carbohydrates (grams)
Strained (Heinz)	4½ oz.	24.0
& apricots, junior (Gerber)	7⁸/₁₀ oz.	47.0
& apricots, junior (Heinz)	7¾ oz.	41.6
& apricots, strained (Gerber)	4⁷/₁₀ oz.	29.2
& apricots, strained (Heinz)	4¾ oz.	23.8
& cherries, junior (Beech-Nut)	7¾ oz.	48.8
& cherries, strained (Beech-Nut)	4¾ oz.	29.3
& pineapple, junior (Gerber)	7⁸/₁₀ oz.	41.7
& pineapple, strained (Gerber)	4⁷/₁₀ oz.	26.4
& raspberries, junior (Beech-Nut)	7¾ oz.	57.8
& raspberries, strained (Beech-Nut)	4¾ oz.	34.6
Apricot with tapioca:		
Junior (Beech-Nut)	7¾ oz.	45.3
Junior (Gerber)	7⁸/₁₀ oz.	44.1
Junior (Heinz)	7¾ oz.	55.0
Strained (Beech-Nut)	4¾ oz.	25.1
Strained (Gerber)	4⁷/₁₀ oz.	26.4
Strained (Heinz)	4¾ oz.	33.3
Banana:		
Strained (Heinz)	4½ oz.	25.0
Pie, junior (Heinz)	7¾ oz.	45.0
Pie, strained (Heinz)	4¾ oz.	25.0
& pineapple, junior (Heinz)	7¾ oz.	40.6
& pineapple, strained (Heinz)	4¾ oz.	25.0
& pineapple with tapioca:		
Junior (Beech-Nut)	7¾ oz.	49.9
Junior (Gerber)	7⁸/₁₀ oz.	44.6
Strained (Beech-Nut)	4¾ oz.	30.2
Strained (Gerber)	4⁷/₁₀ oz.	27.4
Dessert, junior (Beech-Nut)	7¾ oz.	49.7
Pudding, junior (Gerber)	7⁸/₁₀ oz.	48.2
With tapioca:		
Strained (Beech-Nut)	4¾ oz.	28.9
Strained (Gerber)	4⁷/₁₀ oz.	27.4
Bean, green:		
Junior (Beech-Nut)	7¼ oz.	12.5
Strained (Beech-Nut)	4½ oz.	7.8
Strained (Gerber)	4½ oz.	8.5
Strained (Heinz)	4½ oz.	6.4
Creamed with bacon, junior (Gerber)	7½ oz.	19.0

*Prepared as Package Directs

Food and Description	Measure or Quantity	Carbohydrates (grams)
In butter sauce, junior (Beech-Nut)	7¼ oz.	16.8
In butter sauce, strained (Beech-Nut)	4½ oz.	10.2
With potatoes & ham, casserole, toddler (Gerber)	6¹/₅ oz.	17.8
Beef:		
Junior (Beech-Nut)	3½ oz.	.3
Junior (Gerber)	3½ oz.	0.
Strained (Beech-Nut)	3½ oz.	0.
Strained (Gerber)	3½ oz.	0.
Beef & beef broth (Heinz):		
Junior	3½ oz.	0.
Strained	3½ oz.	0.
Beef & beef heart, strained (Gerber)	3½ oz.	.7
Beef dinner:		
Junior (Beech-Nut)	4½ oz.	7.3
Strained (Beech-Nut)	4½ oz.	7.7
& noodles, junior (Beech-Nut)	7½ oz.	15.7
& noodles, junior (Gerber)	7½ oz.	16.7
& noodles, strained (Beech-Nut)	4½ oz.	9.4
& noodles, strained (Gerber)	4½ oz.	9.6
& noodles, strained (Heinz)	4½ oz.	9.3
With vegetables:		
Junior (Gerber)	4½ oz.	7.9
Strained (Gerber)	4½ oz.	8.0
Strained (Heinz)	4¾ oz.	7.1
With vegetables & cereal, junior (Heinz)	4¾ oz.	5.8
Beef lasagna, toddler (Gerber)	6¹/₅ oz.	17.2
Beef liver, strained (Gerber)	3½ oz.	2.0
Beef liver soup, strained (Heinz)	4½ oz.	8.1
Beef stew, toddler (Gerber)	6¹/₅ oz.	15.2
Beet:		
Strained (Gerber)	4½ oz.	11.0
Strained (Heinz)	4½ oz.	12.7
Blueberry buckle (Gerber):		
Junior	7⁸/₁₀ oz.	45.7
Strained	4½ oz.	26.2
Butterscotch pudding (Gerber):		
Junior	7½ oz.	39.7

*Prepared as Package Directs

Food and Description	Measure or Quantity	Carbohydrates (grams)
Strained	4½ oz.	23.3
Caramel pudding (Beech-Nut):		
Junior	7¾ oz.	48.8
Strained	4¾ oz.	29.7
Carrot:		
Junior (Beech-Nut)	7½ oz.	17.6
Junior (Gerber)	7½ oz.	14.9
Junior (Heinz)	7¾ oz.	19.0
Strained (Beech-Nut)	4½ oz.	10.4
Strained (Gerber)	4½ oz.	9.0
Strained (Heinz)	4½ oz.	11.6
& pea, junior (Gerber)	7½ oz.	16.1
In butter sauce (Beech-Nut):		
Junior	7½ oz.	24.2
Strained	4½ oz.	15.0
Cereal, dry:		
Barley (Gerber)	3 T. (7 grams)	5.3
Barley, instant (Heinz)	2 T.	3.9
High protein (Gerber)	3 T. (7 grams)	3.3
High protein, instant (Heinz)	2 T.	3.7
Hi-protein (Beech-Nut)	1 oz.	13.0
Mixed (Beech-Nut)	1 oz.	19.6
Mixed (Gerber)	3 T. (7 grams)	5.3
Mixed (Heinz)	2 T.	4.0
Mixed, honey (Beech-Nut)	1 oz.	20.0
Mixed, with banana (Gerber)	3 T. (7 grams)	5.5
Oatmeal (Beech-Nut)	1 oz.	19.1
Oatmeal (Gerber)	3 T. (7 grams)	4.7
Oatmeal, honey (Beech-Nut)	1 oz.	19.8
Oatmeal, instant (Heinz)	2 T.	3.2
Oatmeal, with banana (Gerber)	3 T. (7 grams)	5.2
Rice (Beech-Nut)	1 oz.	21.7
Rice (Gerber)	3 T. (7 grams)	5.5
Rice, honey (Beech-Nut)	1 oz.	22.5
Rice, instant (Heinz)	2 T.	4.2
Rice, with strawberry (Gerber)	3 T. (7 grams)	5.7
Cereal, or mixed cereal:		
With applesauce & banana:		
Junior (Gerber)	7⁸/₁₀ oz.	40.6
Strained (Gerber)	4⁷/₁₀ oz.	24.4
Strained (Heinz)	4¾ oz.	26.9
With egg yolks & bacon:		
Junior (Beech-Nut)	7½ oz.	17.4

*Prepared as Package Directs

Food and Description	Measure or Quantity	Carbohydrates (grams)
Junior (Gerber)	7½ oz.	15.1
Junior (Heinz)	7½ oz.	15.5
Strained (Beech-Nut)	4½ oz.	10.4
Strained (Gerber)	4½ oz.	9.0
Strained (Heinz)	4½ oz.	10.0
With fruit, strained (Beech-Nut)	4¾ oz.	26.0
High protein with apple & banana, strained (Heinz)	4¾ oz.	25.8
Oatmeal, with applesauce & banana, junior (Gerber)	7$^8/_{10}$ oz.	35.4
Oatmeal with applesauce & banana, strained (Gerber)	4$^7/_{10}$ oz.	20.7
Oatmeal, with fruit, strained (Beech-Nut)	4¾ oz.	20.6
Rice, with applesauce & banana, strained (Gerber)	4$^7/_{10}$ oz.	21.3
Cheese:		
Cottage, creamed with pineapple:		
Junior (Beech-Nut)	7¾ oz.	35.7
Strained (Gerber)	4$^7/_{10}$ oz.	23.3
Cottage, creamed with pineapple juice, strained (Beech-Nut)	4¾ oz.	23.3
Cottage, dessert, with pineapple (Gerber):		
Junior	7$^8/_{10}$ oz.	37.4
Strained	4½ oz.	21.7
Cottage, with banana (Heinz):		
Junior	7¾ oz.	36.3
Strained	4½ oz.	20.9
Cherry vanilla pudding (Gerber):		
Junior	7$^8/_{10}$ oz.	43.3
Strained	4$^7/_{10}$ oz.	29.8
Chicken:		
Junior (Beech-Nut)	3½ oz.	0.
Junior (Gerber)	3½ oz.	.5
Strained (Beech-Nut)	3½ oz.	.4
Strained (Gerber)	3½ oz.	.1
Chicken & chicken broth (Heinz):		
Junior	3½ oz.	0.
Strained	3½ oz.	0.
Chicken dinner:		
Junior (Beech-Nut)	4½ oz.	9.0

*Prepared as Package Directs

Food and Description	Measure or Quantity	Carbohydrates (grams)
Strained (Beech-Nut)	4½ oz.	9.3
Noodle:		
Junior (Beech-Nut)	7½ oz.	15.5
Junior (Gerber)	7½ oz.	17.0
Junior (Heinz)	7½ oz.	15.7
Strained (Beech-Nut)	4½ oz.	9.7
Strained (Gerber)	4½ oz.	10.4
Strained (Heinz)	4½ oz.	9.2
With vegetables:		
Junior (Beech-Nut)	7½ oz.	17.6
Junior (Gerber)	4½ oz.	7.9
Junior (Heinz)	4¾ oz.	5.3
Strained (Beech-Nut)	4½ oz.	10.5
Strained (Gerber)	4½ oz.	7.7
Strained (Heinz)	4¾ oz.	5.8
Chicken soup:		
Junior (Heinz)	7½ oz.	17.6
Strained (Heinz)	4½ oz.	8.9
Cream of, junior (Gerber)	7½ oz.	19.6
Cream of, strained (Gerber)	4½ oz.	12.4
Chicken stew, toddler (Gerber)	6 oz.	15.0
Chicken sticks:		
Junior (Beech-Nut)	2½ oz.	1.6
Junior (Gerber)	2½ oz.	.8
Cookie, animal-shaped (Gerber)	1 cookie (6 grams)	4.3
Cookie, assorted (Beech-Nut)	½ oz.	9.5
Corn, creamed:		
Junior (Gerber)	7½ oz.	29.4
Junior (Heinz)	7½ oz.	34.0
Strained (Beech-Nut)	4½ oz.	26.5
Strained (Gerber)	4½ oz.	18.1
Strained (Heinz)	4½ oz.	20.4
Custard:		
Junior (Beech-Nut)	7¾ oz.	40.5
Junior (Heinz)	7¾ oz.	36.4
Strained (Beech-Nut)	4½ oz.	24.7
Strained (Heinz)	4½ oz.	21.6
Chocolate, junior (Gerber)	7⁸/10 oz.	41.1
Chocolate, strained (Beech-Nut)	4½ oz.	27.8
Chocolate, strained (Gerber)	4½ oz.	24.4
Vanilla, junior (Gerber)	7½ oz.	39.7
Vanilla, strained (Gerber)	4½ oz.	23.4

*Prepared as Package Directs

Food and Description	Measure or Quantity	Carbohydrates (grams)
Egg yolk:		
Strained (Beech-Nut)	3⅓ oz.	1.3
Strained (Gerber)	3³/₁₀ oz.	0.
Strained (Heinz)	3¼ oz.	2.0
& bacon, strained (Beech-Nut)	3⅓ oz.	3.3
& ham, strained (Gerber)	3³/₁₀ oz.	0.
Fruit (Heinz):		
Mixed, & honey, junior	7½ oz.	52.0
Mixed, & honey, with tapioca, strained	4½ oz.	24.7
Fruit dessert:		
Junior (Heinz)	7¾ oz.	50.9
Strained (Heinz)	4½ oz.	30.4
Tropical, junior (Beech-Nut)	7¾ oz.	51.0
With tapioca:		
Junior (Beech-Nut)	7¾ oz.	53.2
Junior (Gerber)	7⁸/₁₀ oz.	49.7
Strained (Beech-Nut)	4¾ oz.	34.4
Strained (Gerber)	4⁷/₁₀ oz.	29.0
Fruit juice:		
Mixed, strained (Beech-Nut)	4¹/₅ fl. oz. (4.4 oz.)	19.0
Mixed, strained (Gerber)	4¹/₅ fl. oz. (4.6 oz.)	18.3
Ham:		
Junior (Gerber)	3½ oz.	.6
Strained (Beech-Nut)	3½ oz.	2.3
Strained (Gerber)	3½ oz.	.7
Ham dinner:		
Junior (Beech-Nut)	4½ oz.	6.4
Strained (Beech-Nut)	4½ oz.	7.8
With vegetables:		
Junior (Gerber)	4½ oz.	8.3
Junior (Heinz)	4¾ oz.	12.5
Strained (Gerber)	4½ oz.	8.5
Strained (Heinz)	4¾ oz.	6.7
Lamb:		
Junior (Beech-Nut)	3½ oz.	0.
Junior (Gerber)	3½ oz.	0.
Strained (Beech-Nut)	3½ oz.	0.
Strained (Gerber)	3½ oz.	0.
& noodles, junior (Beech-Nut)	7½ oz.	18.2
Lamb & lamb broth (Heinz):		
Junior	3½ oz.	0.

*Prepared as Package Directs

Food and Description	Measure or Quantity	Carbohydrates (grams)
Strained	3½ oz.	0.
Liver with liver broth, strained (Heinz)	3½ oz.	0.
Macaroni:		
Alphabets & beef casserole, toddler (Gerber)	6¹/₅ oz.	18.6
& bacon, junior (Beech-Nut)	7½ oz.	20.0
& beef with vegetables, junior (Beech-Nut)	7½ oz.	15.5
With tomato, beef & bacon:		
Junior (Gerber)	7½ oz.	21.9
Junior (Heinz)	7½ oz.	20.6
Strained (Gerber)	4½ oz.	11.9
Strained (Heinz)	4½ oz.	11.6
With tomato sauce, beef & bacon dinner, strained (Beech-Nut)	4½ oz.	11.0
Meat sticks, junior:		
(Beech-Nut)	2½ oz.	.9
(Gerber)	2½ oz.	1.0
Noodles & beef, junior (Heinz)	7½ oz.	16.4
Orange-apple juice, strained:		
(Beech-Nut)	4¹/₅ fl. oz. (4.4 oz.)	23.2
(Gerber)	4¹/₅ fl. oz. (4.6 oz.)	16.3
Orange-apple-banana juice, strained:		
(Gerber)	4¹/₅ fl. oz. (4.6 oz.)	20.2
(Heinz)	4½ fl. oz.	21.8
Orange-apricot juice, strained:		
(Beech-Nut)	4¹/₅ fl. oz. (4.4 oz.)	27.4
(Gerber)	4¹/₅ fl. oz. (4.6 oz.)	18.8
(Heinz)	4½ fl. oz.	17.5
Orange-banana juice, strained (Beech-Nut)	4¹/₅ fl. oz. (4.4 oz.)	28.4
Orange juice, strained:		
(Beech-Nut)	4¹/₅ fl. oz. (4.4 oz.)	14.5
(Gerber)	4¹/₅ fl. oz. (4.6 oz.)	14.5
(Heinz)	4½ fl. oz.	16.2
Orange-pineapple dessert, strained (Beech-Nut)	4¾ oz.	38.5
Orange-pineapple juice, strained:		
(Beech-Nut)	4¹/₅ fl. oz. (4.4 oz.)	24.7

*Prepared as Package Directs

Food and Description	Measure or Quantity	Carbohydrates (grams)
(Gerber)	4¹/₅ fl. oz. (4.6 oz.)	18.6
(Heinz)	4½ fl. oz.	17.5
Orange pudding, strained:		
(Gerber)	4⁷/₁₀ oz.	29.4
(Heinz)	4½ oz.	28.0
Pea:		
Strained (Beech-Nut)	4½ oz.	15.2
Strained (Gerber)	4½ oz.	10.1
Pea, creamed (Heinz):		
Junior	7¾ oz.	24.9
Strained	4½ oz.	12.8
Pea, in butter sauce (Beech-Nut):		
Junior	7¼ oz.	25.2
Strained	4½ oz.	17.0
Peach:		
Junior (Beech-Nut)	7¾ oz.	46.9
Junior (Gerber)	7⁸/₁₀ oz.	44.4
Junior (Heinz)	7½ oz.	60.1
Strained (Beech-Nut)	4¾ oz.	28.3
Strained (Gerber)	4⁷/₁₀ oz.	26.9
Strained (Heinz)	4½ oz.	37.9
Peach cobbler (Gerber):		
Junior	7⁸/₁₀ oz.	47.1
Strained	4⁷/₁₀ oz.	28.5
Peach & honey (Heinz):		
Junior	7½ oz.	37.0
With tapioca, strained	4½ oz.	22.1
Peach Melba (Beech-Nut):		
Junior	7¾ oz.	59.3
Strained	4¾ oz.	36.7
Peach pie (Heinz):		
Junior	7¾ oz.	46.9
Strained	4¾ oz.	28.1
Pear:		
Junior (Beech-Nut)	7½ oz.	38.4
Junior (Gerber)	7⁸/₁₀ oz.	39.4
Junior (Heinz)	7¾ oz.	40.0
Strained (Beech-Nut)	4½ oz.	23.0
Strained (Gerber)	4⁷/₁₀ oz.	24.3
Strained (Heinz)	4½ oz.	23.2
Pear & pineapple:		
Junior (Beech-Nut)	7½ oz.	40.7

*Prepared as Package Directs

Food and Description	Measure or Quantity	Carbohydrates (grams)
Junior (Gerber)	7^8/$_{10}$ oz.	39.5
Junior (Heinz)	7¾ oz.	38.0
Strained (Beech-Nut)	4½ oz.	24.3
Strained (Gerber)	4^7/$_{10}$ oz.	24.6
Strained (Heinz)	4¾ oz.	24.9
Pineapple dessert, strained (Beech-Nut)	4¾ oz.	34.7
Pineapple-grapefruit juice drink, strained (Gerber)	4^1/$_5$ fl. oz. (4.6 oz.)	18.6
Pineapple juice, strained (Heinz)	4½ fl. oz.	16.6
Pineapple-orange dessert (Heinz):		
Junior	7¾ oz.	49.3
Strained	4½ oz.	27.7
Pineapple pie (Heinz):		
Junior	7¾ oz.	49.5
Strained	4¾ oz.	30.8
Plum with tapioca:		
Junior (Beech-Nut)	7¾ oz.	53.0
Junior (Gerber)	7^8/$_{10}$ oz.	53.8
Strained (Beech-Nut)	4¾ oz.	34.4
Strained (Gerber)	4^7/$_{10}$ oz.	32.7
Strained (Heinz)	4½ oz.	31.7
Pork:		
Junior (Beech-Nut)	3½ oz.	1.1
Junior (Gerber)	3½ oz.	0.
Strained (Beech-Nut)	3½ oz.	.4
Strained (Gerber)	3½ oz.	0.
Pork with pork broth, strained (Heinz)	3½ oz.	0.
Potatoes, creamed, with ham, toddler (Gerber)	6 oz.	18.4
Pretzel (Gerber)	1 piece (5 grams)	3.9
Prune-orange juice:		
Strained (Beech-Nut)	4^1/$_5$ fl. oz. (4.4 oz.)	22.8
Strained (Gerber)	4^1/$_5$ fl. oz. (4.6 oz.)	23.6
Strained (Heinz)	4½ fl. oz.	19.9
Prune with tapioca:		
Junior (Beech-Nut)	7¾ oz.	49.3
Junior (Gerber)	7^8/$_{10}$ oz.	49.4
Strained (Beech-Nut)	4¾ oz.	31.1
Strained (Gerber)	4^7/$_{10}$ oz.	29.3
Strained (Heinz)	4¾ oz.	33.7

*Prepared as Package Directs

Food and Description	Measure or Quantity	Carbohydrates (grams)
Raspberry cobbler (Gerber):		
Junior	7⁸/₁₀ oz.	44.4
Strained	4½ oz.	25.2
Spaghetti & meat balls, toddler (Gerber)	6¹/₅ oz.	21.5
Spaghetti, tomato sauce & beef:		
Junior (Beech-Nut)	7½ oz.	20.1
Junior (Gerber)	7½ oz.	27.2
Junior (Heinz)	7½ oz.	26.8
Spaghetti, tomato sauce & meat, strained (Heinz)	4½ oz.	14.6
Spinach, creamed:		
Junior (Gerber)	7½ oz.	14.1
Strained (Gerber)	4½ oz.	8.3
Strained (Heinz)	4½ oz.	8.3
Split pea with bacon, junior (Gerber)	7½ oz.	26.6
Split pea, vegetables & bacon:		
Junior (Heinz)	7½ oz.	23.6
Strained (Heinz)	4½ oz.	13.4
Split pea, vegetables & ham, junior (Beech-Nut)	7½ oz.	23.1
Squash:		
Junior (Beech-Nut)	7½ oz.	16.3
Junior (Gerber)	7½ oz.	13.4
Strained (Beech-Nut)	4½ oz.	9.7
Strained (Gerber)	4½ oz.	8.2
Strained (Heinz)	4½ oz.	10.5
In butter sauce (Beech-Nut):		
Junior	7½ oz.	21.4
Strained	4½ oz.	12.7
Sweet potato:		
Junior (Beech-Nut)	7¾ oz.	31.3
Junior (Gerber)	7⁸/₁₀ oz.	35.9
Strained (Beech-Nut)	4½ oz.	16.9
Strained (Gerber)	4⁷/₁₀ oz.	21.7
Strained (Heinz)	4½ oz.	18.8
In butter sauce (Beech-Nut):		
Junior	7¾ oz.	33.3
Strained	4½ oz.	19.5
Teething biscuit (Gerber)	1 piece (.4 oz.)	8.2
Teething ring, honey (Beech-Nut)	½ oz.	10.7

*Prepared as Package Directs

Food and Description	Measure or Quantity	Carbohydrates (grams)
Tuna with noodles, strained		
(Heinz)	4½ oz.	9.3
Turkey:		
Junior (Beech-Nut)	3½ oz.	.7
Junior (Gerber)	3½ oz.	.1
Strained (Beech-Nut)	3½ oz.	1.0
Strained (Gerber)	3½ oz.	.3
Turkey dinner:		
Junior (Beech-Nut)	4½ oz.	8.4
Strained (Beech-Nut)	4½ oz.	10.8
With rice:		
Junior (Gerber)	7½ oz.	15.9
Strained (Beech-Nut)	4½ oz.	12.7
Strained (Gerber)	4½ oz.	9.7
With rice & vegetables, junior		
(Beech-Nut)	7½ oz.	17.0
With vegetables:		
Junior (Gerber)	4½ oz.	8.3
Strained (Gerber)	4½ oz.	7.8
Strained (Heinz)	4¾ oz.	7.9
Tutti frutti dessert (Heinz):		
Junior	7¾ oz.	44.6
Strained	4½ oz.	25.1
Veal:		
Junior (Beech-Nut)	3½ oz.	0.
Junior (Gerber)	3½ oz.	0.
Strained (Beech-Nut)	3½ oz.	0.
Strained (Gerber)	3½ oz.	0.
Veal dinner:		
Junior (Beech-Nut)	4½ oz.	6.9
Strained (Beech-Nut)	4½ oz.	7.7
With vegetables:		
Junior (Gerber)	4½ oz.	9.4
Junior (Heinz)	4¾ oz.	7.1
Strained (Gerber)	4½ oz.	8.6
Strained (Heinz)	4¾ oz.	6.3
Veal & veal broth (Heinz):		
Junior	3½ oz.	0.
Strained	3½ oz.	0.
Vegetables:		
Garden, strained (Beech-Nut)	4½ oz.	11.3
Garden, strained (Gerber)	4½ oz.	7.9

*Prepared as Package Directs

Food and Description	Measure or Quantity	Carbohydrates (grams)
Mixed, junior (Gerber)	7½ oz.	18.4
Mixed, junior (Heinz)	7½ oz.	20.8
Mixed, strained (Gerber)	4½ oz.	10.9
Vegetables & bacon:		
Junior (Beech-Nut)	7½ oz.	18.0
Junior (Gerber)	7½ oz.	18.7
Junior (Heinz)	7½ oz.	16.3
Strained (Beech-Nut)	4½ oz.	9.7
Strained (Gerber)	4½ oz.	13.0
Strained (Heinz)	4½ oz.	9.0
Vegetables & beef:		
Junior (Beech-Nut)	7½ oz.	15.5
Junior (Gerber)	7½ oz.	14.7
Junior (Heinz)	7½ oz.	17.1
Strained (Beech-Nut)	4½ oz.	10.2
Strained (Gerber)	4½ oz.	8.6
Strained (Heinz)	4½ oz.	8.5
Vegetables & chicken (Gerber):		
Junior	7½ oz.	21.2
Strained	4½ oz.	9.0
Vegetables, dumplings, beef & bacon (Heinz):		
Junior	7½ oz.	16.9
Strained	4½ oz.	10.3
Vegetables, egg noodles & chicken (Heinz):		
Junior	7½ oz.	17.6
Strained	4½ oz.	11.2
Vegetables, egg noodles & turkey, junior (Heinz)	7½ oz.	16.6
Vegetables & ham:		
Junior (Heinz)	7½ oz.	15.4
Strained (Beech-Nut)	4½ oz.	10.5
With bacon, junior (Gerber)	7½ oz.	18.5
With bacon, strained (Gerber)	4½ oz.	9.8
With bacon, strained (Heinz)	4½ oz.	7.3
Vegetables & lamb:		
Junior (Beech-Nut)	7½ oz.	15.5
Junior (Gerber)	7½ oz.	16.2
Junior (Heinz)	7½ oz.	17.4
Strained (Gerber)	4½ oz.	9.9
Strained (Heinz)	4½ oz.	8.1

*Prepared as Package Directs

Food and Description	Measure or Quantity	Carbohydrates (grams)
Vegetables & liver:		
Junior (Beech-Nut)	7½ oz.	16.7
Strained (Beech-Nut)	4½ oz.	10.0
With bacon, junior (Gerber)	7½ oz.	17.9
With bacon, strained (Gerber)	4½ oz.	8.4
Vegetables & turkey:		
Junior (Gerber)	7½ oz.	17.7
Strained (Gerber)	4½ oz.	11.0
Toddler, casserole (Gerber)	6¹/₅ oz.	18.0
Vegetable soup:		
Junior (Beech-Nut)	7½ oz.	18.2
Junior (Heinz)	7½ oz.	20.4
Strained (Beech-Nut)	4½ oz.	11.3
Strained (Heinz)	4½ oz.	10.2
BAC ONION (Lawry's)	1 pkg.	57.1
BAC*OS (General Mills)	1 T.	1.0
BACON:		
Raw (Wilson)	8 oz.	2.4
(Oscar Mayer) 11–14 slices per lb. raw	1 slice (cooked)	.1
(Oscar Mayer) 18–26 slices per lb. raw	1 slice (cooked)	<.1
(Oscar Mayer) 25–30 slices per ¾ lb. raw	1 slice (cooked)	<.1
BACON BITS:		
(French's)	1 oz.	5.7
(McCormick)	1 oz.	7.7
BACON, CANADIAN:		
(Oscar Mayer)	1-oz. slice	0.
(Wilson)	1-oz. slice	<.1
BAGEL:		
Egg	3" dia.	28.0
Water	3" dia.	30.0
BAKING POWDER:		
(Calumet)	1 tsp.	.5
(Royal)	1 tsp.	1.3

*Prepared as Package Directs

Food and Description	Measure or Quantity	Carbohydrates (grams)
BAKON DELITES (Wise):		
Regular	½-oz. bag	0.
Barbecue flavor	½-oz. bag	.3
BANANA:		
Common	1 lb.	68.5
Red	1 lb.	72.2
BANANA CAKE MIX:		
*(Betty Crocker) layer	1 cake	512.4
*(Duncan Hines)	1 cake	490.0
(Pillsbury)	1 oz.	22.7
(Pillsbury) loaf cake	1 oz.	22.6
BANANA PIE:		
Frozen (Mrs. Smith's)	8″ pie	170.0
Frozen (Morton)	14.4-oz. pie	139.8
BANANA PUDDING (Del Monte)	5-oz. can	31.7
BANANA PUDDING & PIE FILLING:		
*Instant (Jell-O)	½ cup	30.5
*Instant (Royal)	½ cup	28.7
*Regular (Jell-O)	½ cup	29.3
*Regular (My-T-Fine)	½ cup	32.6
*Regular (Royal)	½ cup	26.4
BARBECUE DINNER MIX:		
(Hunt's) *Skillet*	2-lb. 1-oz. pkg.	247.1
*Without added fat (Lipton)	1 pkg.	93.6
BARDOLINO WINE (Antinori) 12% alcohol	3 fl. oz.	6.3
BASS	any quantity	0.
B and B LIQUEUR (Julius Wile) 86 proof	1 fl. oz.	5.7
BAVARIAN PIE FILLING (Lucky Leaf)	8 oz.	51.8
BAVARIAN PIE or PUDDING MIX:		
*Cream (My-T-Fine)	½ cup	32.5
*Custard, *Rice-A-Roni*	4 oz.	24.6

*Prepared as Package Directs

Food and Description	Measure or Quantity	Carbohydrates (grams)
BAVARIAN-STYLE BEANS & SPAETZLE (Birds Eye)	10-oz. pkg.	35.4
BEAN, BAKED:		
Canned with brown sugar sauce:		
(B & M) red kidney bean	1 cup	49.7
(B & M) yellow eye bean	1 cup	50.6
(Homemaker's) red kidney bean	1 cup	50.2
Canned in molasses sauce:		
(Heinz)	1 cup	52.8
& brown sugar sauce (Campbell)	1 cup	48.1
Canned with pork:		
(Campbell) Home Style	1 cup	52.0
(Hunt's) *Snack Pack*	5-oz. can	35.3
(Van Camp)	1 cup	41.8
Canned with pork & molasses sauce:		
(B & M) Michigan Pea, New England-style	1 cup	50.8
(Heinz) Boston-style	1 cup	50.8
(Homemaker's) Michigan Pea, New England-style	1 cup	48.8
Canned with pork & tomato sauce:		
(Campbell)	1 cup	42.7
(Heinz)	1 cup	48.5
(Libby's)	1 cup	52.7
Canned with tomato sauce:		
(Heinz) *Campside*	1 cup	51.1
(Heinz) vegetarian	1 cup	48.9
(Van Camp)	1 cup	52.0
BEAN & FRANKFURTER, canned:		
(Campbell) in tomato & molasses sauce	1 cup	35.7
(Heinz)	1 can	38.0
(Van Camp) *Beanie-Weenee*	1 cup	27.6
BEAN & FRANKFURTER DINNER:		
(Banquet)	10 ¾-oz. dinner	70.5
(Morton)	12-oz. dinner	81.3
(Swanson)	11½-oz. dinner	70.1
BEAN, GREEN:		
Fresh, whole	1 lb.	28.3

*Prepared as Package Directs

Food and Description	Measure or Quantity	Carbohydrates (grams)
Canned, cut, solids & liq. (Comstock-Greenwood)	½ cup	4.4
Frozen:		
Cut (Birds Eye)	9-oz. pkg.	15.3
Whole (Birds Eye)	9-oz. pkg.	15.6
French-style (Birds Eye)	9-oz. pkg.	15.3
French-style with sliced mushrooms (Birds Eye)	9-oz. pkg.	16.5
French-style with toasted almonds (Birds Eye)	9-oz. pkg.	18.0
In butter sauce (Green Giant)	9-oz. pkg.	10.2
In mushroom sauce (Green Giant)	10-oz. pkg.	19.8
BEAN, KIDNEY or RED:		
(Sinsheimer)	4 oz.	70.3
Canned solids & liq.	½ cup	21.0
BEAN, LIMA, young:		
Raw, whole	1 lb.	40.1
Raw, without shell	1 lb.	100.2
Canned solids & liq. (Stokely-Van Camp)	½ cup	15.4
Frozen:		
Baby butter beans (Birds Eye)	10-oz. pkg.	70.8
(Birds Eye)	10-oz. pkg.	63.0
In butter sauce (Green Giant)	10-oz. pkg.	47.7
Fordhooks (Birds Eye)	10-oz. pkg.	53.7
BEAN, LIMA (Sinsheimer)	4 oz.	70.0
BEAN, PINTO (Sinsheimer)	4 oz.	70.3
BEAN SALAD:		
(Hunt's) *Snack Pack*	5-oz. can	23.7
(Le Sueur)	1-lb. 1-oz. can	43.5
BEAN, SEMI-MATURE, drained (B & M)	8¾-oz. can	51.8
BEAN SOUP, canned:		
(Manischewitz)	1 can	35.2
*With smoked pork (Heinz)	1 cup	20.1

*Prepared as Package Directs

Food and Description	Measure or Quantity	Carbohydrates (grams)
BEAN SOUP, BLACK:		
(Campbell)	1 can	27.6
(Crosse & Blackwell)	1 can	31.0
BEAN SPROUT:		
Raw, mung	½ lb.	15.0
Raw, soy	½ lb.	12.0
Canned (Mow Sang)	28-oz. can	6.0
BEAN, WHITE, navy or pea		
(Sinsheimer)	4 oz.	70.4
BEAN, YELLOW or WAX:		
Raw	1 lb.	24.0
Canned:		
Golden, whole (Green Giant)	8.5-oz. can	6.0
Cut (Green Giant)	8.5-oz. can	7.2
Frozen, cut (Birds Eye)	9-oz. pkg.	16.2
BEAUJOLAIS WINE, French		
(B & G) 12% alcohol	3 fl. oz.	.1
BEEF	any quantity	0.
BEEFARONI (Chef Boy-Ar-Dee)	40-oz. can	139.5
BEEF BOUILLON/BROTH:		
(Croyden House) instant	1 tsp.	2.2
(Herb-Ox) (Steero)	1 cube	.5
(Herb-Ox) instant	1 packet	.8
(Maggi) (Wyler's)	1 cube or 1 tsp.	.5
(Wyler's) no salt added	1 cube	1.7
BEEF & CABBAGE, casserole		
(Mrs. Paul's)	12-oz. pkg.	27.5
BEEF, CHIPPED:		
(Armour Star)	1 oz.	.0
Cooked (Oscar Mayer)	1 thin slice	.1
Frozen, creamed (Banquet)	5-oz. bag	9.2
BEEF, CHOPPED or DICED		
canned:		
(Armour Star)	12-oz. can	4.4
(Hormel)	12-oz. can	2.0

*Prepared as Package Directs

Food and Description	Measure or Quantity	Carbohydrates (grams)
BEEF DINNER:		
(Banquet)	11-oz. dinner	24.0
(Swanson)	11½-oz. dinner	30.3
(Swanson) 3-course	15-oz. dinner	57.8
Chopped (Banquet)	9-oz. dinner	27.0
Chopped sirloin (Swanson)	10-oz. dinner	40.0
Chopped (Weight Watchers)	18-oz. dinner	6.2
Sliced (Morton) 3-course	1-lb. 1-oz. dinner	60.1
BEEF & EGGPLANT (Mrs. Paul's)	12-oz. pkg.	31.7
BEEF GOULASH:		
Canned (Heinz)	8½-oz. can	20.1
Seasoning mix (Lawry's)	1.7-oz. pkg.	24.1
BEEF & GREEN PEPPER, casserole (Mrs. Paul's)	12-oz. pkg.	31.7
BEEF, GROUND, seasoning mix:		
With onions (Durkee)	1⅛-oz. pkg.	19.9
With onions (French's)	1⅛-oz. pkg.	17.5
BEEF HASH, ROAST (Stouffer's)	11½-oz. pkg.	21.7
BEEF PATTIES, & Burgundy sauce, frozen (Morton House)	4¹/₆-oz. serving	8.9
BEEF PIE:		
(Banquet)	2-lb 4-oz. pie	132.2
(Stouffer's)	10-oz. pie	42.9
(Swanson)	16-oz. pie	56.8
BEEF PUFFS (Durkee)	1 piece	3.1
BEEF, SLICED, with barbecue sauce (Banquet)	5-oz. bag	13.0
BEEF SOUP:		
(Campbell)	1 can	37.6
Barley (Manischewitz)	1 can	22.4
Consommé (Campbell)	1 can	5.2
*Noodle (Heinz)	1 cup	6.7
Vegetable (Manischewitz)	1 can	17.8

*Prepared as Package Directs

Food and Description	Measure or Quantity	Carbohydrates (grams)
BEEF SOUP MIX, noodle (Lipton)		
Cup-a-Soup	1 pkg.	6.4
BEEF STEW:		
(Armour Star)	24-oz. can	38.8
(Austex)	15½-oz. can	31.2
(Bunker Hill)	23-oz. can	28.0
(Heinz)	8½-oz. can	24.2
(Wilson)	15½-oz. can	30.8
Dietetic (Claybourne)	8-oz. can	18.4
Dietetic (Slim-ette)	8-oz. can	22.6
Meatball (Hormel)	1-lb. 8-oz. can	27.9
Frozen:		
Buffet (Banquet)	2-lb. pkg.	82.2
Family (Tom Thumb)	3-lb. 8-oz. tray	97.3
BEEF STEW SEASONING MIX:		
(Durkee)	1 pkg. (1¾-oz.)	22.1
(French's)	1 pkg.	28.5
(Lawry's)	1 pkg.	24.2
BEEF STROGANOFF:		
Canned (Hormel)	1-lb. can	9.5
Mix (Chef Boy-Ar-Dee)	6⅔-oz. pkg.	30.6
Mix (Hunt's) *Skillet*	1-lb. 2-oz. pkg.	94.0
BEER, regular:		
Buckeye, 4.6% alcohol	12 fl. oz.	11.0
Budweiser, 4.9% alcohol	12 fl. oz.	12.3
Budweiser, 3.9% alcohol	12 fl. oz.	11.9
Busch Bavarian, 4.9% alcohol	12 fl. oz.	12.3
Busch Bavarian, 3.9% alcohol	12 fl. oz.	11.9
Gold Medal	12 fl. oz.	9.6
Hamm's	12 fl. oz.	13.3
Knickerbocker, 4.6% alcohol	12 fl. oz.	13.7
Meister Brau Premium, 4.6% alcohol	12 fl. oz.	11.0
Meister Brau Premium Draft, 4.6% alcohol	12 fl. oz.	11.0
Michelob, 4.9% alcohol	12 fl. oz.	12.8
Narragansett, 4.7% alcohol	12 fl. oz.	14.4
North Star, regular	12 fl. oz.	14.9
North Star, 3.2 low gravity	12 fl. oz.	13.6

*Prepared as Package Directs

Food and Description	Measure or Quantity	Carbohydrates (grams)
Pfeifer, regular	12 fl. oz.	14.9
Pfeifer, 3.2 low gravity,	12 fl. oz.	13.6
Rheingold, 4.6% alcohol	12 fl. oz.	13.7
Schlitz	12 fl. oz.	14.7
Schmidt, regular or extra special	12 fl. oz.	14.9
Schmidt, 3.2 low gravity	12 fl. oz.	13.6
Yuengling Premium	12 fl. oz.	15.1
BEER, low carbohydrate:		
Dia-beer	12 fl. oz.	4.2
Dia-beer	7 fl. oz.	2.8
Gablinger's, 4.5% alcohol	12 fl. oz.	.2
Meister Brau Lite, 4.6% alcohol	12 fl. oz.	1.4
BEER, NEAR, *Kingsbury* (Heileman) 0.4% alcohol	12 fl. oz.	15.0
BEET:		
Raw, without tops	1 lb.	31.4
Solids & liq., tiny, whole (Le Sueur)	1-lb. can	36.4
Solids & liq., slices (Libby's)	½ cup	8.1
Frozen, sliced, in orange flavor glaze (Birds Eye)	10-oz. pkg.	44.7
BENEDICTINE LIQUEUR (Julius Wilc) 86 proof	1 fl. oz.	10.3
BIG WHEEL (Hostess)	1 cake	21.6
BISCUIT, egg (Stella D'oro):		
Dietetic	1 piece	6.6
Regular	1 piece	6.9
Roman	1 piece	19.2
Sugared	1 piece	11.0
BISCUIT DOUGH:		
*(Borden) *Gem*	1 biscuit	16.0
(Pillsbury) buttermilk, Tenderflake	1 oz.	11.1
(Pillsbury) *Hungry Jack*, Butter Tastin'	1 oz.	10.4
BISCUIT MIX, *Bisquick* (Betty Crocker)	1 cup	79.4

*Prepared as Package Directs

Food and Description	Measure or Quantity	Carbohydrates (grams)
BITTER LEMON: ·		
(Hoffman)	6 fl. oz.	21.3
(Schweppes)	6 fl. oz.	23.6
BITTER ORANGE (Schweppes)	6 fl. oz.	22.6
BITTERS (Angostura)	1 tsp.	2.1
BLACKBERRY:		
Fresh, with hulls	1 lb.	55.6
Canned, heavy syrup	½ cup	28.9
Canned, low calorie (S and W)		
Nutradiet	4 oz.	11.2
BLACKBERRY PIE:		
(Tastykake)	4-oz. pie	60.1
(Banquet)	5-oz. serving	55.5
BLACKBERRY PIE FILLING, canned:		
(Comstock)	1 cup	108.5
(Lucky Leaf)	8 oz.	62.4
BLACK-EYED PEA, frozen (Birds Eye)	½ cup	15.7
BLOODY MARY MIX (Bar-Tender's)	1 serving	5.7
BLUEBERRY:		
Fresh, untrimmed	1 lb.	63.8
Quick thaw (Birds Eye)	½ cup	28.7
BLUEBERRY PIE:		
(Tastykake)	4-oz. pie	57.8
(Banquet)	5-oz. serving	55.8
(Morton)	20-oz. pie	201.0
(Morton)	46-oz. pie	452.0
(Mrs. Smith's)	8" pie	240.0
(Mrs. Smith's) natural juice	9" pie	364.0
(Mrs. Smith's)	10" pie	420.0
Tart (Pepperidge Farm)	3-oz. pie tart	34.5

*Prepared as Package Directs

Food and Description	Measure or Quantity	Carbohydrates (grams)
BLUEBERRY PIE FILLING:		
(Comstock)	1 cup	82.8
(Lucky Leaf)	8 oz.	61.4
BLUEBERRY TURNOVER, frozen		
(Pepperidge Farm)	1 turnover	32.0
BLUEFISH	any quantity	0.
BOLOGNA:		
All meat (Armour Star)	1-oz. slice	0.
All meat (Hormel)	1 oz.	.5
All meat (Oscar Mayer)	1-oz. slice	.8
Pure beef (Oscar Mayer)	.8-oz. slice	.7
BORSCHT (Manischewitz)	1 cup	17.5
BOSCO (Best Foods)	1 T.	12.9
***BOSTON CREAM PIE,** mix (Betty Crocker)	1 pie	383.2
BOYSENBERRY (S and W) *Nutradiet*	4 oz.	9.8
BOYSENBERRY PIE:		
(Banquet)	5-oz. serving	55.8
(Morton)	20-oz. pie	217.8
BRAINS, all animals	1 lb.	3.6
BRAN BREAKFAST CEREAL:		
Plain:		
All-Bran (Kellogg's)	1 oz.	21.8
Bran Buds (Kellogg's)	1 oz.	21.9
40% bran flakes (Kellogg's)	1 oz.	22.9
40% bran flakes (Post)	1 oz.	21.0
100% bran (Nabisco)	1 oz.	18.6
Raisin bran flakes:		
(Kellogg's)	1 oz.	22.7
(Post)	1 oz.	21.0
Cinnamon (Post)	1 oz.	21.0

*Prepared as Package Directs

Food and Description	Measure or Quantity	Carbohydrates (grams)
BRANDY, FLAVORED:		
Apricot (Bols) 70 proof	1 fl. oz.	7.4
Blackberry (Garnier) 70 proof	1 fl. oz.	7.1
Cherry (Hiram Walker) 70 proof	1 fl. oz.	7.0
Coffee (Leroux) coffee & brandy, 70 proof	1 fl. oz.	8.3
Ginger (Old Mr. Boston) 70 proof	1 fl. oz.	1.0
Peach (Mr. Boston's) peach & brandy, 42 proof	1 fl. oz.	8.0
BRATWURST (Oscar Mayer)	1-oz. slice	.4
BRAUNSCHWEIGER:		
(Oscar Mayer)	1-oz. slice	.2
(Wilson)	1-oz. slice	.7
Liver cheese (Oscar Mayer)	3-oz. slice	.6
BRAZIL NUT, whole	4 oz.	5.9
BREAD:		
Cheese, party (Pepperidge Farm)	6-gram slice	2.7
Cracked-wheat (Pepperidge Farm)	.9-oz. slice	13.0
Daffodil Farm (Wonder)	.8-oz. slice	11.3
Date-nut loaf (Thomas')	1.1-oz. slice	18.5
Finn Crisp	1 piece	4.8
French (Pepperidge Farm)	1" slice	15.8
Glutogen Gluten (Thomas')	.5-oz. slice	6.4
Italian (Pepperidge Farm)	1" slice	16.3
King's Bread (Wasa)	3.5-oz. slice	75.0
Natural Health (Arnold)	.9-oz. slice	10.8
Oatmeal:		
(Arnold)	.8-oz. slice	10.9
(Pepperidge Farm)	.9-oz. slice	12.4
Profile, dark (Wonder)	.8-oz. slice	11.0
Profile, light (Wonder)	.8-oz. slice	11.2
Protogen Protein (Thomas')	.7-oz. slice	8.9
Pumpernickel:		
(Arnold) Jewish	1.4-oz. slice	18.9
(Levy's)	1.1-oz. slice	2.4
(Pepperidge Farm) family	1.2-oz. slice	15.8
(Pepperidge Farm) party	8-gram slice	3.8
(Wonder)	.8-oz. slice	11.0

*Prepared as Package Directs

Food and Description	Measure or Quantity	Carbohydrates (grams)
Raisin:		
Cinnamon (Pepperidge Farm)	.9-oz. slice	13.6
Cinnamon (Thomas')	.8-oz. slice	12.0
Cinnamon (Wonder)	.8-oz slice	13.0
Rite Diet (Thomas')	.7-oz. slice	9.3
Roman Meal	.8-oz. slice	11.2
Rye:		
(Arnold) Melba thin, Jewish	.6-oz. slice	7.8
(Arnold) Jewish, seeded or unseeded	1.2-oz. slice	16.7
(Levy's) with or without caraway	1.1-oz. slice	12.1
(Levy's) Westchester, with or without seeds	1.1-oz. slice	12.1
(Pepperidge Farm) family	1.2-oz. slice	15.7
(Pepperidge Farm) party	6-gram slice	3.0
(Pepperidge Farm) seedless	1.2-oz. slice	15.4
Ry-King (Wasa):		
Brown	1 piece	8.4
Golden	1 piece	6.8
Lite	1 piece	6.2
Seasoned	1 piece	6.8
(Wonder)	.8-oz. slice	10.5
Wheat germ (Pepperidge Farm)	.9-oz. slice	12.2
White:		
(Arnold) Melba thin	.5-oz. slice	7.1
(Arnold) sandwich	.9-oz. slice	11.4
(Pepperidge Farm):		
Large loaf, Calif. only	.8-oz. slice	11.4
Very thin slice, East	.5-oz. slice	7.9
Very thin slice, Mid-west	.6-oz. slice	8.0
Brick Oven (Arnold) 1-lb. loaf	.8-oz. slice	11.0
Hearthstone (Arnold) 1-lb. loaf	.9-oz. slice	12.0
Whole-wheat, *Brick Oven*, 1-lb. loaf	.8-oz. slice	10.0
BREAD, CANNED:		
Banana nut (Dromedary)	½" slice	12.4
Brown, plain (B & M)	½" slice	18.2
Brown with raisins (B & M)	½" slice	17.6
Chocolate nut (Dromedary)	½" slice	14.5
Date & nut (Crosse & Blackwell)	½" slice	12.6
Date & nut (Dromedary)	½" slice	12.8
Orange nut (Dromedary)	½" slice	13.4

*Prepared as Package Directs

Food and Description	Measure or Quantity	Carbohydrates (grams)
BREAD CRUMBS:		
(Old London)	1 cup	97.2
Seasoned (Contadina)	1 cup	77.6
BREAD STICK:		
Cheese or sesame (Keebler)	1 piece	1.8
Dietetic (Stella D'oro)	1 pireciece	6.3
Garlic or salt (Keebler)	1 piece	1.9
Onion (Stella D'oro)	1 piece	6.8
Regular (Stella D'oro)	1 piece	6.6
BREAD STUFFING MIX:		
Corn bread (Pepperidge Farm)	8-oz. pkg.	167.1
Cube (Pepperidge Farm)	7-oz. pkg.	147.0
Herb seasoned (Pepperidge Farm)	8-oz. bag	178.8
BROADBEAN, Italian bean (Birds Eye)	9-oz. pkg.	12.3
BROCCOLI:		
Raw, whole	1 lb.	20.9
Cut (Birds Eye)	10-oz. pkg.	10.8
Spears (Birds Eye)	10-oz. pkg.	10.8
In butter sauce (Green Giant)	10-oz. pkg.	14.1
In cheese sauce (Green Giant)	10-oz. pkg.	16.8
In Hollandaise sauce (Birds ⅜ye)	10-oz. pkg.	9.6
BROTWURST (Oscar Mayer)	3-oz. link	3.1
BRUSSELS SPROUT:		
Raw	1 lb.	34.6
Au gratin, casserole (Green Giant)	10-oz. pkg.	22.5
Baby sprouts (Birds Eye)	10-oz. pkg.	17.1
In butter sauce (Green Giant)	10-oz. pkg.	14.1
BUCKWHEAT GROATS:		
(Pocono)	1 oz.	22.0
Wolff's Kasha (Birkett)	1 oz.	23.3

*Prepared as Package Directs

Food and Description	Measure or Quantity	Carbohydrates (grams)
BUC WHEATS (General Mills)	1 cup	23.4
BULGUR, canned	8 oz.	79.4
BURGUNDY WINE:		
(Italian Swiss Colony-Gold Medal) 12.3% alcohol	3 fl. oz.	.7
(Taylor) 12½% alcohol	3 fl. oz.	Tr.
BURGUNDY WINE, SPARKLING:		
(B & G) 12% alcohol	3 fl. oz.	2.2
(Chanson)	3 fl. oz.	3.6
(Gold Seal) 12% alcohol	3 fl. oz.	2.6
BUTTER:		
Regular	1 stick	.5
Whipped	1 stick	.3
*BUTTER BRICKLE LAYER CAKE MIX (Betty Crocker)	1 cake	430.8
BUTTERSCOTCH MORSELS (Nestlé's)	6-oz. pkg.	102.1
BUTTERSCOTCH PIE (Banquet)	2½-oz. serving	27.0
BUTTERSCOTCH PUDDING:		
Chilled (Breakstone)	5-oz. container	32.5
Chilled (Sealtest)	4 oz.	20.6
(Del Monte)	5-oz. can	32.6
(Hunt's)	5-oz. can	30.3
(Sanna) *Swiss Miss*	5-oz. container	26.0
BUTTERSCOTCH PUDDING or PIE MIX:		
Sweetened:		
*Instant (Jell-O)	½ cup	30.5
*Instant (Royal)	½ cup	28.8
*Regular (Jell-O)	½ cup	29.3
*Regular (My-T-Fine)	½ cup	32.5
*Regular (Royal)	½ cup	32.8
*Low calorie (D-Zerta)	½ cup	4.8

*Prepared as Package Directs

C

CABBAGE, raw:

White	1 lb.	19.3
Red	1 lb.	24.7
Savoy	1 lb.	16.5

CABBAGE, CHINESE or CELERY, raw | 1 lb. | 13.2

CABBAGE, SPOON or WHITE MUSTARD or PAKCHOY, raw | 1 lb. | 12.5

CAKE DECORATOR (Pillsbury) | 1 oz. | 21.0

CAKE ICING (Betty Crocker):

Butterscotch	16.5-oz. can	333.6
Chocolate	16.5-oz. can	300.0
Dark Dutch fudge	16.5-oz. can	296.4
Lemon or vanilla	16.5-oz. can	336.0

CAKE ICING MIX (Betty Crocker):

Cherry, creamy	1 cake's icing	351.6
Coconut-pecan	1 cake's icing	199.2
Coconut, toasted	1 cake's icing	344.4
Orange	1 cake's icing	339.6
Spice	1 cake's icing	350.4
White, fluffy	1 cake's icing	178.8

CAKE MIX:

White:

*(Betty Crocker)	1 cake	426.0
*(Duncan Hines)	1 cake	435.6
(Pillsbury)	1 oz.	21.4
*(Swans Down)	1 cake	434.4

Yellow:

*(Betty Crocker)	1 cake	426.0
*Golden butter (Duncan Hines)	1 cake	444.0
*(Swans Down)	1 cake	433.2

CANDY:

Almonds, candy-coated (Hershey's)	1 oz.	17.2
Almond cluster (Peter Paul)	1³/₁₆-oz. pkg.	19.8

*Prepared as Package Directs

Food and Description	Measure or Quantity	Carbohydrates (grams)
Almond Joy (Peter Paul)	1¾-oz. pkg.	28.1
Baby Ruth (Curtiss)	1 oz.	21.0
Baffle Bar (Cardinet's)	1¾-oz. bar	10.9
Bridge Mix (Nabisco)	1 piece	1.4
Butterfinger (Curtiss)	1 oz.	21.0
Candy corn (Brach's)	1 piece	1.8
Caramel, chocolate or vanilla (Kraft)	1 piece	6.2
Caravelle (Peter Pan)	1½-oz. pkg.	28.5
Cashew crunch, canned (Planters)	1 oz.	14.4
Charleston Chew	10¢ size	26.9
Cherry, chocolate-covered: (Brach's) (Nabisco)	1 piece	13.2
Chocolate bar:		
Milk chocolate:		
(Ghirardelli)	1.1-oz. bar	18.9
(Hershey's)	1 oz.	16.1
Semisweet (Nestlé's)	1 oz.	17.3
Chocolate bar with almonds:		
(Ghirardelli)	1.1-oz. bar	17.6
(Nestlé's)	1 oz.	15.3
Chocolate block, milk (Hershey's)	1 oz.	17.8
Chuckles	1 oz.	23.0
Cluster, peanut (Brach's)	1 piece	7.0
Coconut:		
Bon Bons (Brach's)	1 piece	12.6
Cream egg (Hershey's)	1 oz.	20.4
Fiddle Faddle	1½-oz. packet	34.7
Fudge:		
(Nabisco) *Home Style*	1 piece	13.9
(Tom Houston)	1.5-oz. bar	29.0
Good & Plenty	1 oz.	24.8
Hollywood	1½-oz. bar	28.9
Kisses (Hershey's)	1 piece	2.7
Krackel Bar (Hershey's)	1 oz.	16.6
Licorice Twist (American Licorice Co.):		
Black	1 piece	6.4
Red	1 piece	7.3
Life Savers (Beech-Nut)	1 drop	2.4
Malted Milk balls (Brach's)	1 piece	1.6
Mars Almond Bar (M & M/ Mars)	1 oz.	16.9

*Prepared as Package Directs

Food and Description	Measure or Quantity	Carbohydrates (grams)
Marshmallow (Campfire)	1 oz.	24.9
Mary Jane (Miller)	5¢ size	21.8
Milky Way	1 oz.	17.7
Mint or peppermint:		
Afterdinner (Richardson)	1 oz.	27.0
(Nabisco)	½-oz. piece	12.5
Mounds (Peter Paul)	1⁹/₁₀-oz. pkg.	31.1
M & M's (M & M/Mars):		
Plain chocolate	1 oz.	18.1
Peanut	1 oz.	16.8
Mr. Goodbar (Hershey's)	1 oz.	11.2
$100,000 Bar (Nestlé's)	1 oz.	18.9
Orange slices (Nabisco) *Chuckles*	1 piece	7.2
Peanut, chocolate-covered (Brach's)	1 piece	1.1
Peanut Block bar (Planter's)	1 oz.	14.0
Peanut Butter Cup (Reese's)	1 oz.	15.4
Raisin, chocolate-covered (BB)	5¢ size pkg.	15.4
Sour balls (Bach's)	1 piece	5.7
Spearmint leaves (Quaker City)	1 oz.	26.2
Sugar Daddy (Nabisco):		
Caramel	1-lb. pkg.	398.6
Choco-flavored	.4-oz. piece	10.6
Nugget	.4-oz. piece	10.5
Taffy, salt-water (Brach's)	1 piece	6.8
Tootsie Roll	1¢ size or midgee	5.0
Variety pack (Nabisco) *Chuckles*	2-oz. pack	50.3
CANDY, DIETETIC:		
Almonds, chocolate-covered (Estee)	1 piece	1.6
Chocolate, assorted *Slimtreats*	1 piece	1.3
Chocolate bar, with almonds		
(Estee)	¾-oz. bar	8.7
Chocolate bar, milk (Estee)	¾-oz. bar	9.4
Gum Drops, assorted (Estee)	1 piece	.8
Hard candy, assorted (Estee)	1 piece	3.0
Mint (Estee)	1 piece	1.0
Petit fours (Estee)	1 piece	2.5
TV mix (Estee)	1 piece	.8
CANTALOUPE, whole	1 lb.	17.0
CAPERS (Crosse & Blackwell)	1 T.	1.0

*Prepared as Package Directs

Food and Description	Measure or Quantity	Carbohydrates (grams)
CAP'N CRUNCH:		
(Quaker)	1 oz.	22.8
Crunchberries (Quaker)	1 oz.	23.8
Peanut butter (Quaker)	1 oz.	21.3
*CARAMEL CAKE MIX (Duncan Hines)	1 cake	420.0
CARAMEL PUDDING (My-T-Fine)	5-oz. can	35.1
CARAWAY SEED	1 oz.	12.3
CARNATION INSTANT BREAKFAST:		
Chocolate	1 pkg.	22.6
Coffee	1 pkg.	24.2
Vanilla	1 pkg.	24.4
Special Morning, strawberry	1 pkg.	33.4
CARP	any quantity	0.
CARROT:		
Raw, partially trimmed	1 lb.	36.1
Canned (Stokely-Van Camp)	½ cup	7.4
Frozen:		
Honey glazed (Green Giant)	10-oz. pkg.	19.8
In butter sauce (Green Giant)	10-oz. pkg.	19.8
With brown sugar glaze (Birds Eye)	10-oz. pkg.	50.4
CASABA MELON, whole	1 lb.	14.7
CASHEW NUT:		
Dry roasted (Flavor House)	1 oz.	6.0
Oil roasted (Skippy)	1 oz.	7.8
CATFISH, fillet	any quantity	0.
CATSUP, regular:		
(Bama)	½ pt.	76.8
(Del Monte)	½ pt.	83.2
(Heinz)	½ pt.	60.8
(Hunt's)	½ pt.	92.8
(Stokely-Van Camp)	½ pt.	70.4
CATSUP, dietetic pack (Tillie Lewis)	½ pt.	24.0

*Prepared as Package Directs

Food and Description	Measure or Quantity	Carbohydrates (grams)
CAULIFLOWER:		
Raw, flowerbuds	1 lb.	23.6
(Birds Eye)	10-oz. pkg.	9.6
Au gratin (Stouffer's)	10-oz. pkg.	18.0
In butter sauce (Green Giant)	10-oz. pkg.	8.4
CAULIFLOWER, PICKLED		
(Smucker's)	1 bud	5.5
CAVIAR, STURGEON:		
Pressed	1 oz.	1.4
Whole	1 oz.	.9
CELERY, fresh, whole	1 lb.	13.3
CERTS (Warner-Lambert)	1 piece	1.5
CERVELAT, dry or soft	1 oz.	.5
CHABLIS WINE:		
(B & G) 12% alcohol	3 fl. oz.	.1
(Chanson) 11½% alcohol	3 fl. oz.	6.3
(Great Western)	3 fl. oz.	1.7
CHAMPAGNE:		
(Bollinger)	3 fl. oz.	3.6
(Great Western) brut, 12.5% alcohol	3 fl. oz.	3.2
(Great Western) extra dry, 12.5% alcohol	3 fl. oz.	4.5
(Lejon) pink, 12% alcohol	3 fl. oz.	2.6
(Mogen David) 12% alcohol	3 fl. oz.	8.9
(Mumm's) extra dry, 12% alcohol	3 fl. oz.	5.6
(Veuve Clicquot) 12½% alcohol	3 fl. oz.	.6
CHARD, Swiss, raw	1 lb.	19.2
CHEERIOS (General Mills)	1 oz.	20.2
CHEESE:		
American or cheddar, natural:		
(Foremost Blue Moon)	1-oz. slice	Tr.
(Kraft)	1 oz.	.6
Cheddar (Sealtest)	1 oz.	.6

*Prepared as Package Directs

Food and Description	Measure or Quantity	Carbohydrates (grams)
Grated (Kraft)	1 oz.	8.4
Shredded (Kraft)	1 oz.	.6
Sharp cheddar, *Wispride*	1 T.	1.5
American or cheddar, process:		
(Borden)	¾-oz. slice	1.2
(Kraft) (Sealtest)	1 oz.	.5
Bleu or Blue:		
(Frigo) (Kraft)	1 oz.	.5
Wispride	1 oz.	3.2
Blufort (Borden)	1¼-oz. pkg.	.7
Brick (Kraft) process	1 oz.	.4
Camembert (Borden) (Kraft)	1 oz.	.5
Caraway (Kraft)	1 oz.	.6
Colby (Borden) (Kraft)	1 oz.	.6
Cottage, creamed, unflavored:		
(Borden)	8-oz. container	6.6
(Kraft)	8-oz. container	7.2
California (Breakstone)	8-oz. container	4.8
Light n' Lively (Sealtest)	1 cup	5.6
Low fat (Breakstone)	8-oz. container	7.9
Tangy or tiny curd (Breakstone)	8-oz. container	4.8
Cottage, creamed, flavored:		
Chive (Sealtest)	1 cup	4.7
Pineapple (Sealtest)	1 cup	16.1
Spring Garden Salad (Sealtest)	1 cup	6.7
Cottage, uncreamed:		
Pot (Borden)	8-oz. pkg.	6.1
Skim milk (Breakstone)	8-oz. container	1.6
Cream cheese:		
Plain:		
Philadelphia (Kraft)	1 oz.	.9
Philadelphia, imitation		
(Kraft)	1 oz.	1.9
Flavored, chive (Borden)	1 oz.	.6
Flavored, whipped (Kraft):		
Bacon & horseradish	1 oz.	.7
Smoked salmon	1 oz.	1.7
Edam (House of Gold) (Kraft)	1 oz.	.3
Gjetost (Kraft)	1 oz.	13.0
Gouda, baby (Foremost Blue Moon)	1 oz.	Tr.
Gruyère (Borden) *Swiss Knight*	1 oz.	.5
Liederkranz (Borden)	1 oz.	.4

*Prepared as Package Directs

Food and Description	Measure or Quantity	Carbohydrates (grams)
Monterey Jack (Borden)	1 oz.	.6
Monterey Jack (Frigo) (Kraft)	1 oz.	.4
Mozzarella:		
(Borden)	1 oz.	.8
Skim, pizza (Kraft)	1 oz.	.3
Muenster (Borden)	1 oz.	.7
Old English (Kraft)	1 oz.	.5
Parmesan, grated (Buitoni)	1 oz.	.8
Parmesan & Romano, grated		
(Borden)	1 oz.	.2
Pimento American (Kraft)	1 oz.	.4
Pizza (Frigo)	1 oz.	.3
Port du Salut (Foremost Blue		
Moon)	1 oz.	Tr.
Provolone (Frigo) (Kraft)	1 oz.	.5
Ricotta (Sierra)	1 oz.	1.3
Roquefort (Borden)	1 oz.	.6
Swiss, domestic:		
Natural (Borden) (Kraft)		
(Sealtest)	1 oz.	.5
Process:		
(Borden)	1-oz. slice	.9
(Borden)	¾-oz. slice	.7
Swiss, imported, natural (Borden)	1 oz.	.5
CHEESE CAKE (Mrs. Smith's)	8″ cake	140.0
*CHEESE CAKE MIX:		
(Jell-O)	1 cake including crust	251.2
(Royal) *No-Bake*	9″ cake including crust	255.2
CHEESE FOOD:		
American, slices (Kraft)	1 oz.	2.4
Links (Kraft) *Handi-Snack,* bacon, garlic, jalapeño, *Nippy, Smokelle*	1 oz.	2.2
Loaf, *Pizzalone* (Kraft)	1 oz.	.5
Pimento, slices (Kraft)	1 oz.	2.5
Swiss (Borden)	1 oz.	1.7
Swiss (Kraft)	1 oz.	2.3

*Prepared as Package Directs

Food and Description	Measure or Quantity	Carbohydrates (grams)
CHEESE PIE, pineapple (Mrs. Smith's)	8″ pie	218.4
CHEESE PUFF (Durkee)	1 piece	2.9
CHEESE SOUFFLE (Stouffer's)	12-oz. pkg.	84.6
CHEESE SPREAD:		
(Borden) *Vera Sharp*	1 oz.	1.8
Bacon (Kraft) *Squeez-A-Snak*	1 oz.	.5
Blue (Borden) *Vera Blue*	1 oz.	.6
Cheez Whiz (Kraft)	1 oz.	1.7
Neufchâtel, clam (Kraft) *Party-Snacks*	1 oz.	.8
Onion, French (Nabisco) *Snack Mate*	1 tsp.	.4
Velveeta (Kraft)	1 oz.	2.6
CHEESE STRAW, frozen (Durkee)	1 piece	1.2
CHERRY:		
Sour:		
Fresh	1 lb.	52.5
Canned, water pack (Stokely-Van Camp)	½ cup	12.2
Sweet:		
Fresh	1 lb.	71.0
Canned, heavy syrup:		
With pits, Royal Anne (Del Monte)	½ cup	28.1
Pitted (Del Monte)	½ cup	23.2
Canned, dietetic pack, pitted:		
(Blue Boy)	4 oz.	10.4
(Tillie Lewis)	½ cup	14.7
Frozen (Birds Eye)	½ cup	30.8
***CHERRY CAKE** (Duncan Hines)	1 cake	417.6
CHERRY, CANDIED (Liberty)	1 oz.	22.6
CHERRY HEERING (Hiram Walker) 49 proof	1 fl. oz.	10.0
CHERRY, MARASCHINO (Liberty)	1 average cherry	1.9

*Prepared as Package Directs

CHERRY PIE:
  (Hostess) — 4½-oz. pie — 56.0
  Frozen:
    (Morton) — 20-oz. pie — 214.2
    (Mrs. Smith's) — 8″ pie — 260.0
    Tart (Pepperidge Farm) — 3-oz. pie tart — 34.3

CHERRY PIE FILLING:
  (Comstock) — 1 cup — 84.6
  (Lucky Leaf) — 8 oz. — 58.2

CHERRY SOFT DRINK:
  Sweetened:
    (Canada Dry) — 6 fl. oz. — 24.0
    (Clicquot Club) (Cott) (Mission) — 6 fl. oz. — 23.0
    (Dr. Brown's) (Key Food)
      (Nedick's) (Waldbaum) — 6 fl. oz. — 20.1
    (Fanta) (Hoffman) — 6 fl. oz. — 21.9
    (Shasta) — 6 fl. oz. — 22.2
    (Yoo-Hoo) — 6 fl. oz. — 18.0
    High-protein (Yoo-Hoo) — 6 fl. oz. — 24.6
    (Yukon Club) — 6 fl. oz. — 21.5
  Unsweetened or low calorie:
    (Clicquot Club) (Cott) (Dr.
      Brown's) (Hoffman) (Key
      Food) (Mission) (Waldbaum)
      (Yukon Club) — 6 fl. oz. — .4
    (No-Cal) — 6 fl. oz. — 0.
    (Shasta) — 6 fl. oz. — .1

CHERRY TURNOVER (Pepperidge
Farm) — 3.3-oz. turnover — 30.3

CHESTNUT, in shell — 4 oz. — 38.7

CHEWING GUM:
  Bazooka, bubble — 5¢ size — 21.2
  Beech-Nut — 1 stick — 2.3
  Spearmint (Wrigley's) — 1 stick — 2.2

CHIANTI WINE:
  (Antinori) 12½% alcohol — 3 fl. oz. — 6.3
  (Italian Swiss Colony-Gold
    Medal) 12.1% alcohol — 3 fl. oz. — 1.4

*Prepared as Package Directs

Food and Description	Measure or Quantity	Carbohydrates (grams)
CHICKEN, raw	any quantity	0.
CHICKEN A LA KING:		
Canned (Richardson & Robbins)	1 cup	14.4
Frozen (Banquet)	5-oz. bag	9.0
CHICKEN CACCIATORE (Hormel)	1-lb. can	8.2
CHICKEN, CANNED, plain	any quantity	0.
CHICKEN, CREAMED (Stouffer's)	11½-oz. pkg.	16.2
CHICKEN DINNER:		
Noodle (Heinz)	8½-oz. can	18.9
Noodle (Lynden Farms)	14-oz. jar	31.8
(Weight Watchers)	10-oz. dinner	6.3
Boneless chicken (Swanson)		
Hungry Man	19-oz. dinner	63.7
Chicken & dumplings:		
Buffet (Banquet)	2-lb. pkg.	110.8
(Morton)	12-oz. dinner	30.7
(Morton) 3-course	1-lb. 5-oz. dinner	90.7
(Tom Thumb)	3-lb. 8-oz. tray	112.6
Creole (Weight Watchers)	12-oz. luncheon	10.2
Fried:		
(Banquet)	11-oz. dinner	48.2
(Morton)	11-oz. dinner	37.2
(Morton) 3-course	1-lb. 1-oz. dinner	73.2
(Swanson)	11½-oz. dinner	46.6
(Swanson) 3-course	15-oz. dinner	62.6
With shoestring potato		
(Swanson)	25-oz. pkg.	135.5
CHICKEN DIP (Durkee)	1 pkg.	27.8
CHICKEN FRICASSEE:		
Canned (College Inn)	1 cup	14.8
Canned (Richardson & Robbins)	1 cup	15.1
CHICKEN, FRIED (Banquet)	2-lb. chicken	92.0
CHICKEN LIVER PUFF (Durkee)	1 piece	3.1

*Prepared as Package Directs

Food and Description	Measure or Quantity	Carbohydrates (grams)
CHICKEN & NOODLES:		
(Banquet) buffet	2-lb. pkg.	61.2
Escalloped (Stouffer's)	11½-oz. pkg.	35.9
CHICKEN PIE:		
(Banquet)	2-lb. 4-oz. pie	132.8
(Stouffer's)	10-oz. pkg.	44.2
(Swanson) deep dish	16-oz. pie	55.5
CHICKEN PUFF (Durkee)	1 piece	3.0
CHICKEN SOUP:		
Broth:		
(Campbell)	1 can	1.8
(College Inn)	1 cup	.1
*Dietetic (Claybourne)	8 oz.	0.
Cream of (Heinz) *Great American*	1 cup	9.0
Noodle (Manischewitz)	1 can	8.4
Rice (Campbell)	1 can	11.2
*Vegetable (Heinz)	1 cup	9.3
CHICKEN SOUP MIX:		
Noodle (Lipton) *Cup-a-Soup*	1 pkg.	5.9
With chicken (Lipton) *Cup-a-Soup*	1 pkg.	5.8
CHICKEN SPREAD:		
(Swanson)	5-oz. can	2.0
(Underwood)	4¾-oz. can	5.0
CHICK PEA or GARBANZO, dry	1 lb.	276.7
CHICORY, WITLOOF, Belgian or French endive	1 lb.	12.8
CHILI or CHILI CON CARNE:		
Canned with beans:		
(Armour Star)	15½-oz. can	59.3
(Austex)	15½-oz. can	53.6
(Wilson)	15½-oz. can	52.8
Canned without beans:		
(Armour Star)	15½-oz. can	25.5
(Austex)	15½-oz. can	24.7
(Wilson)	15½-oz. can	25.4

*Prepared as Package Directs

Food and Description	Measure or Quantity	Carbohydrates (grams)
*CHILI DOG SAUCE MIX		
(McCormick)	.9-oz. serving	4.0
CHILI SAUCE:		
(Del Monte)	½ pt.	73.6
(Heinz)	½ pt.	60.8
(Hunt's)	½ pt.	78.4
(Stokely-Van Camp)	½ pt.	56.0
CHILI SEASONING MIX:		
Chili-O (French's)	1¾-oz. pkg.	23.8
(Lawry's)	1.6-oz. pkg.	23.6
CHINESE DINNER (Chun King):		
Egg Foo Young	11-oz. dinner	53.0
Shrimp Chow Mein	11-oz. dinner	50.0
CHITTERLINGS (Hormel)	1-lb. 2-oz. can	.5
CHOCOLATE, BAKING:		
Bitter:		
(Baker's)	1-oz. sq.	7.7
Pre-melted, *Choco-Bake*	1-oz. packet	10.2
(Hershey's)	1 oz.	6.3
Sweetened:		
Chips, milk (Hershey's)	1 oz.	16.7
Chips, semisweet (Baker's)	¼ cup	28.5
Chips, semisweet (Ghirardelli)	⅓ cup	35.6
Chips, semisweet (Hershey's)	1 oz.	17.7
German's, sweet (Baker's)	1 oz.	16.9
Morsels, milk (Nestlé's)	1 oz.	18.0
Morsels, semisweet (Nestlé's)	6-oz. pkg.	108.4
Morsels, semisweet (Nestlé's)	1 oz.	18.1
Semisweet (Baker's)	1-oz. sq.	16.7
CHOCOLATE CAKE:		
(Sara Lee)	1 oz.	16.0
Fudge (Pepperidge Farm)	18-oz. cake	260.4
German (Sara Lee)	1 oz.	12.0
Golden (Pepperidge Farm)	18-oz. cake	261.6
CHOCOLATE CAKE MIX:		
*Chocolate malt layer (Betty Crocker)	1 cake	429.6

*Prepared as Package Directs

Food and Description	Measure or Quantity	Carbohydrates (grams)
*Deep chocolate (Duncan Hines)	1 cake	410.4
*German chocolate (Swans Down)	1 cake	429.6
CHOCOLATE DRINK (Borden)	9½-fl.-oz. can	32.1
CHOCOLATE DRINK MIX, *Quik* (Nestlé's)	2 heaping tsps.	14.4
CHOCOLATE ICE CREAM:		
(Borden) 9.5% fat	¼ pt.	16.9
(Meadow Gold) 10% fat	¼ pt.	16.5
(Prestige) French	¼ pt.	18.0
(Sealtest)	¼ pt.	17.3
CHOCOLATE PIE:		
(Mrs. Smith's)	8″ pie	200.0
Tart (Pepperidge Farm)	3-oz. pie tart	35.2
Velvet nut (Kraft)	16¾-oz. pie	182.4
CHOCOLATE PUDDING:		
Chilled (Breakstone)	5-oz. container	35.5
Canned (Hunt's)	5-oz. can	30.5
CHOCOLATE PUDDING or PIE FILLING MIX:		
Regular:		
*(My-T-Fine)	½ cup	31.3
*(Royal)	½ cup	31.7
*Instant (Jello-O)	½ cup	33.4
*Low calorie (D-Zerta)	½ cup	11.0
CHOCOLATE RENNET MIX:		
(Junket)	1 tablet	.2
CHOCOLATE SOFT DRINK:		
Sweetened:		
(Clicquot Club) (Cott) (Mission)	6 fl. oz.	22.0
(Hoffman) *Cocoa Cooler*	6 fl. oz.	22.3
(Hoffman) (Yukon Club)	6 fl. oz.	21.9
(Yoo Hoo)	6 fl. oz.	18.0
(Yoo Hoo) high protein	6 fl. oz.	24.6
Low calorie:		
(Clicquot Club) (Cott) (Mission)	6 fl. oz.	.2

*Prepared as Package Directs

Food and Description	Measure or Quantity	Carbohydrates (grams)
(Hoffman) (Shasta)	6 fl. oz.	.2
(No-Cal)	6 fl. oz.	0.
CHOCO-NUT SUNDAE CONE		
(Sealtest)	2½ fl. oz.	21.5
CHOP SUEY:		
Canned:		
Chicken (Mow Sang)	20-oz. can	14.0
Pork (Mow Sang)	20-oz. can	14.0
Frozen, beef (Banquet)	2-lb. pkg.	43.8
CHOW CHOW (Crosse &		
Blackwell)	1 T.	1.0
CHOW MEIN:		
Beef (Chun King) *Divider-Pak*	28-oz. can	44.0
Chicken (Chun King) *Divider-Pak*	28-oz. can	48.0
Pork (Chun King) *Divider-Pak*	28-oz. can	44.0
Frozen, chicken:		
(Banquet)	2-lb. pkg.	49.2
(Chun King)	15 oz. pkg.	24.0
CHUTNEY, *Major Grey's*	1 T.	13.1
CITRON, CANDIED (Liberty)	1 oz.	22.6
CLACKERS (General Mills)	1 oz.	22.1
CLAM:		
Hard or round	1 lb.	6.1
Soft	1 lb.	5.3
Chopped & minced, solids &		
liq. (Doxsee)	8 oz.	6.4
CLAM CHOWDER:		
Manhattan:		
(Crosse & Blackwell)	13-oz. can	25.8
(Snow)	8 oz.	7.8
New England:		
(Crosse & Blackwell)	13-oz. can	20.6
(Snow)	8 oz.	16.9
CLAM COCKTAIL (Sau-Sea)	4-oz. jar	19.1

*Prepared as Package Directs

Food and Description	Measure or Quantity	Carbohydrates (grams)
CLAM JUICE (Snow)	8 oz.	1.6
CLARET WINE (Gold Seal) 12% alcohol	3 fl. oz.	.4
CLORETS	1 piece	1.3
CLUB SODA SOFT DRINK, regular or dietetic, any brand	6 fl. oz.	0.
COCOA, dry:		
(Droste)	1 T.	2.9
(Hershey's)	1-oz. packet	13.1
COCOA KRISPIES (Kellogg's)	1 oz.	25.2
COCOA MIX:		
(Nestlé's) *EverReady*	3 heaping tsps.	19.6
Instant, rich chocolate (Carnation)	1-oz. pkg.	20.4
COCOA PEBBLES (Post)	1 oz.	25.0
COCOA PUFFS (General Mills)	1 oz.	25.2
COCONUT:		
Whole	1 lb.	22.2
Dried:		
Angel Flake (Baker's)	½ cup	14.8
Cookie (Baker's)	½ cup	23.2
Crunchies (Baker's)	½ cup	20.6
Premium shred (Baker's)	½ cup	18.2
Southern-style (Baker's)	½ cup	14.8
COCONUT CAKE (Pepperidge Farm)	18-oz. cake	276.0
***COCONUT CAKE MIX** (Duncan Hines)	1 cake	420.0
COCONUT PIE:		
Cream:		
(Morton)	14.4-oz. pie	148.4
(Mrs. Smith's)	8″ pie	190.0

*Prepared as Package Directs

Food and Description	Measure or Quantity	Carbohydrates (grams)
Custard:		
(Morton)	20-oz. pie	166.2
(Mrs. Smith's)	8″ pie	190.0
*COCONUT PUDDING MIX:		
Cream, instant (Jell-O)	½ cup	29.0
Toasted, instant (Royal)	½ cup	27.3
COD, raw	any quantity	0.
COFFEE:		
*Regular (Maxwell House)	¾ cup	.4
Instant, *Nescafé*	1 slightly rounded tsp.	.7
*Decaffeinated, *Sanka*, instant	¾ cup	.9
Freeze-dried, *Taster's Choice*	1 slightly rounded tsp.	.7
COFFEE CAKE:		
(Drake's) large	11-oz. cake	186.8
Blueberry ring (Sara Lee)	1 oz.	15.0
Danish, apple (Morton)	13.5-oz. cake	166.6
Danish, apple (Sara Lee)	1 oz.	11.0
Danish, cherry (Sara Lee)	1 oz.	11.0
Danish pecan twist (Morton)	12-oz. cake	149.4
Lemon ring (Drake's)	13-oz. cake	217.3
Melt-A-Way (Morton)	13-oz. cake	184.8
Pecan ring (Drake's)	13-oz. cake	210.8
Raspberry ring (Drake's)	13-oz. cake	199.6
*COFFEE CAKE MIX (Aunt Jemima)	1 cake	177.0
COLA SOFT DRINK:		
Sweetened:		
(Canada Dry) Jamaica	6 fl. oz.	19.2
(Clicquot Club) (Cott) (Mission)	6 fl. oz.	20.0
Coca-Cola	6 fl. oz.	18.5
(Dr. Brown's) (Hoffman) (Nedick's) (Waldbaum)	6 fl. oz.	20.1
(Key Food) regular	6 fl. oz.	19.4
(Key Food) cherry	6 fl. oz.	18.8
Mr. Cola	6 fl. oz.	20.3
Pepsi-Cola	6 fl. oz.	19.7

*Prepared as Package Directs

Food and Description	Measure or Quantity	Carbohydrates (grams)
RC with a twist (Royal Crown)	6 fl. oz.	20.5
(Yukon Club)	6 fl. oz	20.4
(Royal Crown) (Shasta)	6 fl. oz.	19.4
Low calorie:		
(No-Cal) (Shasta) *Tab*	6 fl. oz.	<.1
(Clicquot Club) (Cott) (Mission)	6 fl. oz.	.1
Diet Pepsi-Cola, sugar-free	6 fl. oz.	<.1
Diet Rite, sugar-free	6 fl. oz.	Tr.
(Dr. Brown's) (Hoffman)		
(Key Food) (Waldbaum)		
(Yukon Club)	6 fl. oz.	.2
RC Cola, sugar-free	6 fl. oz.	Tr.
COLD DUCK WINE (Italian Swiss Colony-Private Stock) 12% alcohol	3 fl. oz.	4.3
COLLARDS:		
Raw	1 lb.	32.7
Frozen, chopped (Birds Eye)	10-oz. pkg.	13.5
COLLINS MIX (Bar-Tender's)	1 serving	17.4
CONCENTRATE (Kellogg's)	1 oz.	15.3
CONCORD WINE (Mogen David) 12% alcohol	3 fl. oz.	16.0
CONSOMME MADRILENE (Crosse & Blackwell)	1 can	4.8
COOKIE:		
Almond crescent (Nabisco)	1 piece	5.0
Almond toast, Mandel (Stella D'oro)	1 piece	9.6
Angelica Goodies (Stella D'oro)	1 piece	14.6
Anginetti (Stella D'oro)	1 piece	2.4
Animal Cracker:		
(Nabisco) *Barnum's*	1 piece	2.0
(Sunshine)	1 piece	1.7
Anisette sponge (Stella D'oro)	1 piece	10.0
Anisette toast (Stella D'oro)	1 piece	7.8

*Prepared as Package Directs

Food and Description	Measure or Quantity	Carbohydrates (grams)
Applesauce (Sunshine)	1 piece	11.9
Arrowroot (Sunshine)	1 piece	3.0
Assortment:		
(Stella D'oro) *Lady Stella*	1 piece	5.0
(Sunshine) *Lady Joan*	1 piece	5.8
Aunt Sally (Sunshine)	1 piece	19.7
Bana-Bee (Nabisco)	1¾-oz. pkg.	31.4
Big Treat (Sunshine)	1 piece	26.6
Bordeaux (Pepperidge Farm)	1 piece	5.1
Breakfast Treats (Stella D'oro)	1 piece	15.0
Brown edge wafers (Nabisco)	1 piece	4.1
Brownie:		
(Drake's) Junior	⅔-oz. cake	10.0
(Hostess) 2 to pkg.	1 piece	15.5
(Tastykake)	2¼-oz. pkg.	34.0
Chocolate nut (Pepperidge Farm)	1 piece	6.3
Peanut butter (Tastykake)	1¾-oz. pkg.	32.0
Pecan fudge (Keebler)	1 piece	13.9
Brussels (Pepperidge Farm)	1 piece	4.6
Butter:		
(Nabisco)	1 piece	3.6
(Sunshine)	1 piece	3.5
Buttercup (Keebler)	1 piece	3.6
Butterscotch Fudgies (Tastykake)	1¾-oz. pkg.	35.0
Capri (Pepperidge Farm)	1 piece	9.7
Cardiff (Pepperidge Farm)	1 piece	2.5
Cherry Coolers (Sunshine)	1 piece	4.5
Chinese almond (Stella D'oro)	1 piece	21.5
Chocolate or chocolate-covered:		
Como (Stella D'oro)	1 piece	16.8
Creme (Wise)	1 piece	4.9
Peanut bars (Nabisco) *Ideal*	1 piece	10.3
Pinwheels (Nabisco)	1 piece	20.9
Snaps (Nabisco)	1 piece	2.7
Snaps (Sunshine)	1 piece	2.4
Wafers (Nabisco) *Famous*	1 piece	4.7
Chocolate chip:		
(Keebler) old fashioned	1 piece	11.0
(Nabisco)	1 piece	4.5
(Nabisco) *Chips Ahoy*	1 piece	7.5
(Nabisco) *Family Favorites*	1 piece	4.5
(Nabisco) snaps	1 piece	3.4

*Prepared as Package Directs

Food and Description	Measure or Quantity	Carbohydrates (grams)
(Pepperidge Farm)	1 piece	6.2
(Sunshine) *Chip-A-Roos*	1 piece	7.7
(Tastykake) *Choc-O-Chip*	1¾-oz. pkg.	34.8
Cinnamon:		
Crisp (Keebler)	1 piece	2.7
Spice, vanilla sandwich		
(Nabisco) *Crinkles*	1⅝-oz. pkg.	33.4
Sugar (Pepperidge Farm)	1 piece	7.0
Toast (Sunshine)	1 piece	2.3
Coconut:		
Bar (Nabisco)	1 piece	6.3
Bar (Sunshine)	1 piece	6.2
Chocolate chip (Nabisco)	1 piece	9.0
Chocolate chip (Sunshine)	1 piece	9.7
Chocolate drop (Keebler)	1 piece	8.5
Coconut Kiss (Tastykake)	1¾-oz. pkg.	33.2
Jumble (Drake's)	1 piece	10.6
Commodore (Keebler)	1 piece	10.1
Como Delight (Stella D'oro)	1 piece	18.3
Cowboys and Indians (Nabisco)	1 piece	1.8
Cream Lunch (Sunshine)	1 piece	7.3
Creme Wafer Stick (Dutch Twin)	1 piece	5.9
Creme Wafer Stick (Nabisco)	1 piece	5.9
Cup Custard (Sunshine)	1 piece	9.3
Devil's Food Cake (Nabisco)	1 piece	9.8
Dixie Vanilla (Sunshine)	1 piece	13.1
Dresden (Pepperidge Farm)	1 piece	10.0
Egg Jumbo (Stella D'oro)	1 piece	7.6
Fig bar:		
(Keebler)	1 piece	14.4
(Nabisco) *Fig Newtons*	1 piece	11.2
(Sunshine)	1 piece	9.2
Fortune (Chun King)	1 piece	4.6
Fruit, iced (Nabisco)	1 piece	13.5
Fudge:		
(Sunshine)	1 piece	9.4
Chip (Pepperidge Farm)	1 piece	6.7
Fudge Stripes (Keebler)	1 piece	7.5
Gingersnap:		
(Keebler)	1 piece	4.3
(Nabisco) old fashioned	1 piece	5.4
(Sunshine)	1 piece	4.4

*Prepared as Package Directs

Food and Description	Measure or Quantity	Carbohydrates (grams)
Zu Zu (Nabisco)	1 piece	3.1
Golden Bars (Stella D'oro)	1 piece	16.0
Golden Fruit (Sunshine)	1 piece	14.4
Hermit bar, frosted (Tastykake)	2-oz. pkg.	60.8
Home Plate (Keebler)	1 piece	9.9
Hydrox (Sunshine)	1 piece	7.1
Jan Hagel (Keebler)	1 piece	6.7
Keebies (Keebler)	1 piece	7.1
Lemon:		
(Sunshine)	1 piece	9.8
Jumble rings (Nabisco)	1 piece	11.0
Lemon Coolers (Sunshine)	1 piece	4.5
Nut crunch (Pepperidge Farm)	1 piece	6.4
Snaps (Nabisco)	1 piece	3.1
Lido (Pepperidge Farm)	1 piece	10.0
Lisbon (Pepperidge Farm)	1 piece	3.3
Macaroon:		
Almond (Tastykake)	2-oz. pkg.	35.1
Coconut (Nabisco) Bake Shop	1 piece	12.1
Sandwich (Nabisco)	1 piece	9.5
Margherite (Stella D'oro)	1 piece	10.6
Marquisette (Pepperidge Farm)	1 piece	5.0
Marshmallow:		
Fancy Crests (Nabisco)	1 piece	10.4
Mallowmars (Nabisco)	1 piece	8.7
Mallo Puff (Sunshine)	1 piece	12.2
Minarets (Nabisco)	1 piece	5.7
Puffs (Nabisco)	1 piece	12.8
Sandwich (Nabisco)	1 piccc	5.7
Twirls (Nabisco)	1 piece	21.9
Milano (Pepperidge Farm)	1 piece	7.2
Milano, mint (Pepperidge Farm)	1 piece	8.4
Mint sandwich (Nabisco) Mystic	1 piece	10.6
Molasses & Spice (Sunshine)	1 piece	11.9
Naples (Pepperidge Farm)	1 piece	3.7
Nassau (Pepperidge Farm)	1 piece	9.2
Oatmeal:		
(Keebler) old fashioned	1 piece	11.7
(Nabisco)	1 piece	12.3
(Sunshine)	1 piece	8.9
Iced (Sunshine)	1 piece	11.6
Irish (Pepperidge Farm)	1 piece	7.1

*Prepared as Package Directs

Food and Description	Measure or Quantity	Carbohydrates (grams)
Peanut butter (Sunshine)	1 piece	10.5
Raisin (Nabisco) *Bake Shop*	1 piece	11.5
Raisin (Pepperidge Farm)	1 piece	7.5
Raisin bar (Tastykake)	2¼-oz. pkg.	47.6
Old Country Treats (Stella D'oro)	1 piece	7.1
Orleans (Pepperidge Farm)	1 piece	3.5
Peach-apricot pastry (Stella D'oro)	1 piece	5.0
Peanut & peanut butter:		
Bars, cocoa-covered (Nabisco)		
Crowns	1 piece	10.0
Caramel logs (Nabisco) *Heydays*	1 piece	13.4
Creme patties (Nabisco)	1 piece	3.9
Creme patties, cocoa-covered		
(Nabisco) *Fancy*	1 piece	6.4
Patties (Sunshine)	1 piece	4.2
Sandwich (Nabisco) *Nutter*		
Butter	1 piece	9.2
Pecan Sandies (Keebler)	1 piece	9.2
Penguins (Keebler)	1 piece	14.0
Pirouette (Pepperidge Farm)	1 piece	4.5
Pitter Patter (Keebler)	1 piece	10.9
Pizzelle, Carolines (Stella D'oro)	1 piece	6.7
Raisin, fruit biscuit (Nabisco)	1 piece	12.3
Rich 'n Chips (Keebler)	1 piece	8.9
Rochelle (Pepperidge Farm)	1 piece	9.6
Sandwich, creme:		
Cameo (Nabisco)	1 piece	10.5
Chocolate chip (Nabisco)	1 piece	9.1
Chocolate fudge:		
(Keebler)	1 piece	13.0
(Nabisco) *Cookie Break*	1 piece	7.0
Orbit (Sunshine)	1 piece	7.0
Oreo (Nabisco)	1 piece	7.3
Oreo & Swiss (Nabisco)	1 piece	7.0
Pride (Nabisco)	1 piece	7.3
Social Tea (Nabisco)	1 piece	7.2
Swiss (Nabisco)	1 piece	6.6
(Tom Houston)	1 piece	8.4
Vanilla (Keebler)	1 piece	11.1
Vanilla (Nabisco)	1 piece	7.0
Vienna Finger (Sunshine)	1 piece	10.5
Sesame, Regina (Stella D'oro)	1 piece	6.9

*Prepared as Package Directs

Food and Description	Measure or Quantity	Carbohydrates (grams)
Shortbread or shortcake:		
(Nabisco) *Dandy*	1 piece	7.7
(Pepperidge Farm)	1 piece	8.3
Lorna Doone (Nabisco)	1 piece	5.1
Pecan (Nabisco)	1 piece	9.0
Scotties (Sunshine)	1 piece	5.0
Striped (Nabisco)	1 piece	6.8
Vanilla (Tastykake)	2¼-oz. pkg.	43.8
Social Tea Biscuit (Nabisco)	1 piece	3.5
Spiced wafers (Nabisco)	1 piece	7.4
Sprinkles (Sunshine)	1 piece	11.4
Sugar cookies:		
(Keebler) old fashioned	1 piece	12.4
(Pepperidge Farm)	1 piece	7.0
(Sunshine)	1 piece	11.9
Brown (Nabisco) *Family Favorite*	1 piece	3.0
Brown (Pepperidge Farm)	1 piece	6.9
Rings (Nabisco)	1 piece	10.7
Sugar wafer:		
(Nabisco) *Biscos*	1 piece	2.5
(Sunshine)	1 piece	6.6
Krisp Kreem (Keebler)	1 piece	3.7
Lemon (Sunshine)	1 piece	6.5
Swedish Kreme (Keebler)	1 piece	12.2
Tahiti (Pepperidge Farm)	1 piece	8.6
Toy (Sunshine)	1 piece	2.1
Vanilla creme (Wise)	1 piece	5.0
Vanilla snap (Nabisco)	1 piece	2.3
Vanilla wafer:		
(Keebler)	1 piece	2.6
(Nabisco) *Nilla*	1 piece	2.9
(Sunshine) small	1 piece	2.2
Venice (Pepperidge Farm)	1 piece	6.3
Waffle creme (Dutch Twin)	1 piece	6.1
Waffle creme (Nabisco) *Biscos*	1 piece	6.0
Yum Yums (Sunshine)	1 piece	10.4
COOKIE, DIETETIC:		
Apple pastry (Stella D'oro)	1 piece	13.6
Assorted (Estee)	1 piece	4.8
Chocolate & vanilla wafer (Estee)	1 piece	3.2
Vanilla filled wafer (Estee)	1 piece	3.2

*Prepared as Package Directs

Food and Description	Measure or Quantity	Carbohydrates (grams)
COOKIE DOUGH, refrigerated (Pillsbury):		
Brownie	1 oz.	7.3
Chocolate chip	1 oz.	17.0
Peanut butter	1 oz.	16.0
COOKIE MIX:		
Brownie:		
*"Cake like," family size (Duncan Hines)	1 pan	482.4
*Fudge, chewy, family size (Duncan Hines)	1 pan	475.2
Fudge (Pillsbury)	1 oz.	21.7
*German chocolate (Betty Crocker)	1½" sq.	12.0
Toll House (Nestlé's)	1 oz.	20.1
COOL 'N CREAMY (Birds Eye)	½ cup	27.7
CORN:		
In husk	1 lb.	36.1
Husk removed	1 lb.	55.1
Canned, regular pack:		
Vacuum pack, *Niblets*	12-oz. can	57.8
Country style (Green Giant)	8.5-oz. can	40.0
Cream style (Green Giant)	8.5-oz. can	45.8
Canned, dietetic pack (Blue Boy)	4 oz.	16.0
Frozen:		
(Birds Eye)	1 ear	21.7
Niblet Ears	1 ear	35.0
Cream style (Green Giant)	10-oz. pkg.	45.4
In butter sauce, *Niblets*	10-oz. pkg.	45.4
Kernel (Birds Eye)	½ cup	17.8
CORNBREAD (Aunt Jemima) corn sticks	3 pieces	19.2
CORNBREAD MIX:		
*(Aunt Jemima)	1 cornbread	207.0
(Pillsbury) *Ballard*	1 oz.	19.2
CORN CHEX	1 oz.	24.2

*Prepared as Package Directs

Food and Description	Measure or Quantity	Carbohydrates (grams)
CORNED BEEF:		
Raw	any quantity	0.
Canned (Armour Star)	12-oz. can	0.
Packaged (Vienna)	1 oz.	.1
CORNED BEEF HASH:		
(Armour Star)	15½-oz. can	36.0
(Austex)	15-oz. can	45.5
(Wilson)	15½-oz. can	31.6
CORNED BEEF SPREAD		
(Underwood)	4½-oz. can	1.3
CORN FLAKES:		
Country (General Mills)	1 oz.	24.3
(Kellogg's) (Ralston)	1 oz.	24.3
(Van Brode)	1 oz.	24.2
CORN FRITTER (Mrs. Paul's)	12-oz. pkg.	123.3
CORNMEAL MIX (Aunt Jemima/ Quaker)	¼ cup	19.7
CORN SOUFFLE (Stouffer's)	12-oz. pkg.	57.0
CORNSTARCH (Argo) (Kingsford's) (Duryea's)	1 T.	8.3
CORN TOTAL (General Mills)	1 oz.	24.3
COUNT CHOCULA (General Mills)	1 oz.	24.5
CRAB:		
Steamed, whole	1 lb.	1.1
Steamed, meat only	1 lb.	2.3
Canned:		
(Del Monte) Alaska King	7½-oz. can	3.6
(Icy Point) (Pillar Rock)	7½-oz. can	2.3
Frozen (Ship Ahoy) King Crab	8-oz. pkg.	.5
CRAB APPLE, whole, fresh	1 lb.	74.3
CRAB CAKE (Mrs. Paul's)	10-oz. pkg.	62.3
CRAB COCKTAIL (Sau-Sea)	4-oz. jar	18.4

*Prepared as Package Directs

Food and Description	Measure or Quantity	Carbohydrates (grams)
CRAB NEWBURG (Stouffer's)	12-oz. pkg.	13.6
CRAB SOUP (Crosse & Blackwell)	1 can	16.6
CRACKER:		
American Harvest (Nabisco)	1 piece	2.0
Arrowroot biscuit (Nabisco)	1 piece	3.5
Bacon flavored thins (Nabisco)	1 piece	1.2
Bacon Nips	1 oz.	15.6
Bacon rinds (Wonder)	1 oz.	0.
Bacon toast (Keebler)	1 piece	2.0
Bugles (General Mills)	15 pieces	7.5
Butter thins (Nabisco)	1 piece	2.4
Cheese flavored:		
Cheese'n Cracker (Kraft)	4 crackers & ¾ oz. cheese	.7
Cheese Nips (Nabisco)	1 piece	.7
Chee·Tos	1 oz.	14.9
Cheez Doodles (Old London)	1⅛-oz. bag	18.5
Cheez-Its (Sunshine)	1 piece	.6
Cheez Waffles (Old London)	1 piece	1.3
Che-zo (Keebler)	1 piece	.6
Ritz (Nabisco)	1 piece	1.9
Shapies (Nabisco)	1 piece	.8
Thins (Pepperidge Farm)	2 pieces	3.5
Thins, dietetic (Estee)	1 piece	.9
Tid-Bit (Nabisco)	1 piece	.6
Toast (Keebler)	1 piece	1.9
Twists (Nalley)	1 oz.	14.2
Twists (Wonder)	1 oz.	14.7
Chicken in a Biskit (Nabisco)	1 piece	1.2
Chippers (Nabisco)	1 piece	1.8
Chipsters (Nabisco)	1 piece	.3
Clam flavored crisps (Snow)	1 oz.	14.9
Club (Keebler)	1 piece	2.0
Corn Capers (Wonder)	1 oz.	15.4
Corn cheeze (Tom Houston)	10 pieces	1.9
Corn chips:		
Cornetts	1 oz.	16.3
Fritos	1 oz.	14.8
Korkers (Nabisco)	1 piece	.9
(Old London)	1¾-oz. bag	27.3

*Prepared as Package Directs

Food and Description	Measure or Quantity	Carbohydrates (grams)
(Wise)	1¾-oz. bag	27.6
(Wonder)	1 oz.	14.8
Barbecue (Wise)	1¾-oz. bag	27.5
Corn Diggers (Nabisco)	1 piece	.5
Crown Pilot (Nabisco)	1 piece	12.4
Dipsy Doodles (Old London)	1¾-oz. bag	26.4
Doo Dads (Nabisco)	1 piece	.3
Escort (Nabisco)	1 piece	2.7
Flings (Nabisco)	1 piece	.6
Goldfish (Pepperidge Farm):		
Cheddar or Parmesan cheese	10 pieces	3.3
Lightly salted, pizza, onion, sesame garlic	10 pieces	3.6
Pretzel	10 pieces	5.0
Graham:		
(Nabisco)	1 piece	5.4
Chocolate or cocoa-covered:		
(Keebler) *Deluxe*	1 piece	5.6
(Nabisco)	1 piece	7.0
(Nabisco) *Fancy*	1 piece	9.0
(Nabisco) *Pantry*	1 piece	8.5
Sweet-Tooth (Sunshine)	1 piece	6.4
Sugar-honey coated (Nabisco) *Honey Maid*	1 piece	5.3
Hi-Ho (Sunshine)	1 piece	2.1
Milk lunch (Nabisco) *Royal Lunch*	1 piece	7.9
Munchos	1 oz.	14.5
Onion flavored:		
Crisps (Snow)	1 oz.	15.9
French (Nabisco)	1 piece	1.6
Funyuns (Frito-Lay)	1 oz.	18.9
Meal Mates (Nabisco)	1 piece	3.4
Onyums (General Mills)	30 pieces	7.7
Rings (Old London)	½-oz. bag	10.4
Rings (Wise)	½-oz. bag	11.1
Rings (Wonder)	1 oz.	19.5
Thins (Pepperidge Farm)	1 piece	2.0
Toast (Keebler)	1 piece	2.1
OTC (Original Trenton Cracker)	1 piece	4.4
Oyster:		
(Keebler)	1 piece	.2
Dandy (Nabisco)	1 piece	.5

*Prepared as Package Directs

Food and Description	Measure or Quantity	Carbohydrates (grams)
Mini (Sunshine)	1 piece	.6
Oysterettes (Nabisco)	1 piece	.6
Peanut butter 'n cheez crackers (Kraft)	4 crackers & ¾ oz. peanut butter	13.4
Peanut butter sandwich:		
Cheese crackers (Wise)	1 piece	3.4
Toasted crackers (Wise)	1 piece	3.7
Pizza Spins (General Mills)	32 pieces	8.0
Pizza Wheels (Wise)	¾-oz. bag	16.1
Potato crisps (General Mills)	16 pieces	7.5
Ritz, plain (Nabisco)	1 piece	2.1
Rye thins (Pepperidge Farm)	1 piece	2.0
Rye toast (Keebler)	1 piece	2.2
Rye wafers (Nabisco) *Meal Mates*	1 piece	3.4
Ry-Krisp:		
Seasoned	1 whole cracker	4.5
Traditional	1 whole cracker	4.8
Saltine:		
Flavor-Kist, any kind	1 piece	2.2
Krispy (Sunshine)	1 piece	2.0
Premium (Nabisco)	1 piece	2.0
Zesta (Keebler)	1 piece	2.0
Sea toast (Keebler)	1 piece	11.1
Sesame:		
(Sunshine) *La Lanne*	1 piece	1.8
Buttery flavored (Nabisco)	1 piece	1.9
Wafer (Keebler)	1 piece	2.0
Wafer (Nabisco) *Meal Mates*	1 piece	3.2
Sesa Wheat (Austin's)	1 piece	3.7
Sip 'n Chips (Nabisco)	1 piece	1.0
Sociables (Nabisco)	1 piece	1.3
Soda:		
(Nabisco) *Premium*	1 piece	2.0
(Sunshine)	1 piece	3.3
Soya (Sunshine) *La Lanne*	1 piece	1.9
Star Lites (Wise)	1 cup	9.9
Swedish rye wafer (Keebler)	1 piece	3.8
Taco tortilla chips (Wonder)	1 oz.	15.9
Tortilla chips (Frito-Lay) *Doritos*	1 oz.	18.3
Tortilla chips (Old London)	1½-oz. bag	27.8
Tortilla chips (Wonder)	1 oz.	17.2

*Prepared as Package Directs

Food and Description	Measure or Quantity	Carbohydrates (grams)
Town House	1 piece	2.0
Triangle Thins (Nabisco)	1 piece	1.1
Triscuit (Nabisco)	1 piece	3.0
Twigs (Nabisco)	1 piece	1.6
Uneeda Biscuit (Nabisco)	1 piece	3.7
Wafer-ets (Hol-Grain):		
Rice	1 piece	2.5
Wheat	1 piece	1.4
Waldorf, low salt (Keebler)	1 piece	2.4
Waverly wafer (Nabisco)	1 piece	2.6
Wheat chips (General Mills)	12 pieces	7.8
Wheat thins (Nabisco)	1 piece	1.2
Wheat toast (Keebler)	1 piece	2.0
Whistles (General Mills)	17 pieces	8.0
White thins (Pepperidge Farm)	1 piece	2.0
Whole-wheat, natural (Froumine)	1 piece	7.5
CRACKER CRUMBS, graham:		
(Keebler)	3 oz.	64.1
(Nabisco)	9″ pie shell	100.3
CRACKER MEAL:		
(Keebler) Zesty	3 oz.	61.5
Unsalted (Nabisco)	1 cup	67.9
CRANAPPLE (Ocean Spray):		
Regular	½ cup	22.9
Low calorie	½ cup	4.7
CRANBERRY, fresh, (Ocean Spray)	1 lb.	47.2
CRANBERRY JUICE COCKTAIL (Ocean Spray):		
Regular	½ cup	19.7
Low calorie	½ cup	6.3
CRANBERRY SAUCE:		
Jellied (Ocean Spray)	4 oz.	42.9
Whole berry (Ocean Spray)	4 oz.	44.3
CRANPRUNE (Ocean Spray)	½ cup	20.1
CRAYFISH, in shell, raw	1 lb.	.7

*Prepared as Package Directs

Food and Description	Measure or Quantity	Carbohydrates (grams)
CREAM:		
Half & half, 10.5% fat (Sealtest)	½ pt.	10.2
Light, 18% fat (Sealtest)	½ pt.	9.6
Heavy whipping, 36% fat (Sealtest)	½ pt.	8.0
Sour:		
(Breakstone)	8-oz. container	8.4
Half & half (Sealtest)	½ pt.	8.0
Imitation, *Sour Treat* (Delite)	½ pt.	12.8
***CREAM OF RICE**	4 oz.	17.9
CREAM or CREME SOFT DRINK:		
Sweetened:		
(Canada Dry) vanilla	6 fl. oz.	24.1
(Clicquot Club) (Cott) (Mission)	6 fl. oz.	22.0
(Dr. Brown's) (Key Food)		
(Nedick's) (Waldbaum)	6 fl. oz.	20.9
(Fanta)	6 fl. oz.	24.2
(Hoffman) (Shasta) (Yukon Club)	6 fl. oz.	21.3
Low calorie:		
(Clicquot Club) (Cott) (Mission)	6 fl. oz.	.5
(Dr. Brown's) (Hoffman) (Key		
Food)(Waldbaum)(Yukon Club)	6 fl. oz.	.2
(No-Cal)	6 fl. oz.	<.1
(Shasta)	6 fl. oz.	<.1
CREAM SUBSTITUTE:		
Coffee-mate (Carnation)	1 packet	1.7
Cremora (Borden)	1 tsp.	1.1
Pream	1 tsp.	1.1
CREAM OF WHEAT, dry:		
Instant or quick	1 oz.	21.2
Regular	1 oz.	21.7
CREME DE CACAO LIQUEUR		
(Bols) 54 proof	1 fl. oz.	11.8
CREME DE MENTHE LIQUEUR		
(Garnier) 60 proof	1 fl. oz.	15.3
CRESS, GARDEN, raw	1 lb.	17.7
CUCUMBER, whole	1 lb.	14.8

*Prepared as Package Directs

Food and Description	Measure or Quantity	Carbohydrates (grams)
CUPCAKE:		
Chocolate (Tastykake)	1 cupcake	33.0
Chocolate, cream-filled (Drake's)	1 cupcake	25.6
Devil's food cake (Hostess) 12 to pkg.	1 cupcake	22.5
Orange (Hostess) 12 to pkg.	1 cupcake	23.7
Raisin Snack (Drake's)	2¼-oz. cake	41.8
CUPCAKE MIX (Flako)	1 pkg.	254.4
CURAÇAO LIQUEUR (Hiram Walker) 60 proof	1 fl. oz.	11.8
CURRANT:		
Fresh	1 lb.	53.2
Dried (Del Monte)	½ cup	54.2
CURRY POWDER (Crosse & Blackwell)	1 T.	3.9
CUSTARD, chilled (Sealtest)	4 oz.	24.3
CUSTARD PUDDING MIX (Lynden Farms)	4-oz. pkg.	69.2

D

Food and Description	Measure or Quantity	Carbohydrates (grams)
DAIQUIRI COCKTAIL:		
Cocktail (Hiram Walker) 52.5 proof	3 fl. oz.	12.0
Cocktail (National Distillers) *Duet*, 12% alcohol	8-fl.-oz. can	24.0
Mix (Bar-Tender's)	1 serving	17.2
DANDELION GREENS, raw	1 lb.	41.7
DANISH-STYLE VEGETABLES (Birds Eye)	10-oz. pkg.	22.8
DATE, dry:		
Chopped (Dromedary)	1 cup	114.2
Pitted (Dromedary)	1 cup	112.3

*Prepared as Package Directs

Food and Description	Measure or Quantity	Carbohydrates (grams)
DESSERT CUP (Del Monte):		
Pudding 'n apricot	5-oz. container	34.9
Pudding 'n peach	5-oz. container	35.5
Pudding 'n pineapple	5-oz. container	34.6
DEVIL DOG (Drake's)	1.6-oz. cake	24.5
DEVIL'S FOOD CAKE (Pepperidge Farm)	1 cake	282.0
DEVIL'S FOOD CAKE MIX:		
*(Duncan Hines)	1 cake	420.0
*(Swans Down)	1 cake	423.6
Red devil (Pillsbury)	1 oz.	21.5
DING DONG (Hostess) 12 to pkg.	1 piece	21.0
DIP:		
Bacon & horseradish:		
(Breakstone)	2 T.	1.3
(Kraft) *Teez*	1 oz.	1.6
Blue cheese (Sealtest) *Dip 'n Dressing*	1 oz.	1.5
Clam:		
(Kraft) *Teez*	1 oz.	1.5
& lobster (Borden)	1 oz.	1.7
Jalapeño bean (Fritos)	1 oz.	4.1
Onion (Sealtest)	1 oz.	2.2
DIP MIX:		
Bacon-onion (Fritos)	1 pkg.	7.2
Bleu cheese (Fritos)	1 pkg.	8.1
Chili con queso (Fritos)	1 pkg.	7.5
Green onion (Fritos)	1 pkg.	10.8
Green onion (Lawry's)	1 pkg.	10.6
Guacamole (Lawry's)	1 pkg.	5.5
Toasted onion (Fritos)	1 pkg.	10.0
Toasted onion (Lawry's)	1 pkg.	9.8
DISTILLED LIQUOR, any proof	1 fl. oz.	
DOUGHNUT:		
(Hostess) 10 to pkg.	1 piece	18.2
Powdered (Morton)	1 piece	9.2

*Prepared as Package Directs

Food and Description	Measure or Quantity	Carbohydrates (grams)
DRAMBUIE LIQUEUR, 80 proof (Hiram Walker)	1 fl. oz.	11.0
DR. BROWN'S CEL-RAY TONIC:		
Regular	6 fl. oz.	16.5
Low calorie	6 fl. oz.	.2
DR. PEPPER:		
Regular	6 fl. oz.	17.4
Sugar free	6 fl. oz.	.4
DUCK, ready-to-cook	any quantity	0.

E

Food and Description	Measure or Quantity	Carbohydrates (grams)
EGG, CHICKEN, raw:		
Whole, medium	1 egg	.4
Whole, jumbo	1 egg	.6
EGG FOO YOUNG (Chun King)	12-oz. pkg.	21.8
EGG NOG:		
(Borden) 4.7% fat	½ cup	16.3
(Meadow Gold) 6% fat	½ cup	25.5
(Sealtest) 8% butterfat	½ cup	17.3
With alcohol (Old Mr. Boston) 30 proof	1 fl. oz.	4.5
EGGPLANT:		
Fried sticks (Mrs. Paul's)	7-oz. pkg.	57.3
Parmesan (Mrs. Paul's)	11-oz. pkg.	47.3
EGG ROLL:		
Chicken (Chun King)	½-oz. roll	3.2
Shrimp (Chun King)	½-oz. roll	3.8
EGGSTRA (Tillie Lewis)	1 large egg	2.2
ENCHILADA:		
Beef (Banquet)	2-lb. pkg.	136.0
With rice (Swanson)	9⅝-oz. pkg.	45.9
ENCHILADA DINNER:		
Beef:		
(Banquet)	12-oz. dinner	61.0

*Prepared as Package Directs

Food and Description	Measure or Quantity	Carbohydrates (grams)
(Patio) 5-compartment	13-oz. dinner	93.0
Cheese:		
(Banquet)	12½-oz. dinner	58.2
(Patio) 5-compartment	12-oz. dinner	55.0
ENCHILADA MIX (Lawry's)	1.6-oz. pkg.	27.3
ENDIVE, CURLY, raw	1 lb.	16.4

F

Food and Description	Measure or Quantity	Carbohydrates (grams)
FARINA, cream, dry (H-O)	1 cup	134.3
FAT, COOKING, any brand	any quantity	0.
FIG:		
Fresh	1 lb.	92.1
Candied (Bama)	1 T.	9.6
Canned:		
(Del Monte)	½ cup	27.4
Unsweetened (Diet Delight)	½ cup	18.2
Dried (Del Monte)	1 cup	96.4
FIG JUICE, *RealFig*	½ cup	15.8
FILBERT or HAZELNUT, whole	1 lb.	34.9
FISH CAKE, thins (Mrs. Paul's)	10-oz. pkg.	71.5
FISH & CHIPS:		
(Gorton)	1-lb. pkg.	78.0
(Swanson)	5-oz. pkg.	28.4
FISH DINNER:		
With French fries (Swanson)	9¾-oz. dinner	41.4
With green beans & peach (Weight Watchers)	18-oz. dinner	21.9
With pineapple chunks (Weight Watchers)	9½-oz. luncheon	17.2
FISH FILLETS (Gorton)	8-oz. pkg.	20.0
FISH PUFFS (Gorton)	8-oz. pkg.	18.0

*Prepared as Package Directs

Food and Description	Measure or Quantity	Carbohydrates (grams)
FISH STICK, breaded, fried (Mrs. Paul's)	14-oz. pkg.	72.6
FLOUNDER, raw	any quantity	0.
FLOUR:		
Buckwheat, dark	1 cup	70.6
Rye, light	1 cup	78.7
Soybean	1 cup	28.5
Wheat:		
Aunt Jemima, self-rising	1 cup	83.2
Gold Medal (Betty Crocker):		
Regular	1 cup	100.7
Better-for-bread	1 cup	98.4
Self-rising	1 cup	100.5
Wondra	1 cup	100.8
Presto, self-rising	1 cup	84.3
Softasilk (Betty Crocker)	1 cup	88.4
FRANKFURTER or WIENER:		
(Armour Star) all meat	1.6-oz. frankfurter	0.
(Oscar Mayer) all meat	1.6-oz. frankfurter	1.3
(Oscar Mayer) pure beef	1.6-oz. frankfurter	1.4
(Wilson) skinless, all meat	1.6-oz. frankfurter	.8
Canned (Hormel)	12-oz. can	2.4
FRANKS-N-BLANKETS (Durkee)	1 piece	1.0
FRENCH TOAST (Aunt Jemima)	1 slice	13.9
FRESCA	6 fl. oz.	<.1
FROG LEGS	any quantity	0.
FROOT LOOPS (Kellogg's)	1 oz.	24.8
FROSTED RICE KRINKLES (Post)	1 oz.	25.0
FROSTED SHAKE (Borden)	9¼-fl.-oz. can	43.0
FROSTY O's (General Mills)	1 oz.	24.0
FROZEN DESSERT:		
Charlotte Freeze (Borden):		
Chocolate	1 pt.	69.3

*Prepared as Package Directs

Food and Description	Measure or Quantity	Carbohydrates (grams)
Vanilla	1 pt.	63.0
Chocolate (SugarLo):		
4.6% fat, ice milk	1 pt.	60.9
10.8% fat, ice cream	1 pt.	61.2
Coffee (SugarLo):		
4% fat, ice milk	1 pt.	57.6
10% fat, ice cream	1 pt.	57.9
Strawberry (SugarLo):		
3.6% fat, ice milk	1 pt.	57.6
9% fat, ice cream	1 pt.	57.9
Vanilla-coated ice cream or ice milk bar (SugarLo)	2½-oz. bar	9.3
FRUIT COCKTAIL:		
Canned, heavy syrup:		
(Hunt's)	½ cup	23.9
(Dole)	½ cup	24.4
Canned, unsweetened (Tillie Lewis)	½ cup	11.4
FRUIT CUP, solids & liquid (Del Monte):		
Fruit cocktail	5¼-oz. container	28.5
Mixed fruit	5¼-oz. container	27.4
Peaches, diced	5¼-qz. container	29.5
Pineapple, in its own juice	4¼-oz. container	17.9
FRUIT, MIXED:		
Dried (Del Monte)	1 cup	118.1
Quick thaw (Birds Eye)	½ cup	28.4
FRUIT SALAD:		
Chilled (Kraft)	4 oz.	13.3
Canned:		
(Del Monte) fruits for salad	½ cup	21.4
Unsweetened (S and W) *Nutradiet*	4 oz.	10.3
FUDGE CAKE MIX:		
Chocolate (Pillsbury)	1 oz.	22.1
*Marble (Duncan Hines)	1 cake	420.0
Sour cream (Pillsbury)	1 oz.	21.2
FUDGE ICE BAR (Sealtest)	2½-fl.-oz. bar	18.6

*Prepared as Package Directs

Food and Description	Measure or Quantity	Carbohydrates (grams)

G

Food and Description	Measure or Quantity	Carbohydrates (grams)
GARLIC, whole	2 oz.	15.4
GARLIC SPREAD (Lawry's)	1 T.	1.2
GATORADE	6 fl. oz.	16.0
GAZPACHO SOUP (Crosse & Blackwell)	13-oz. can	13.6
GEFILTE FISH:		
(Manischewitz) 1-lb. jar	1 piece	2.3
(Mother's) 1-lb. jar	1 piece	2.3
GELATIN (Knox)	1 envelope	0.
***GELATIN DESSERT POWDER:**		
(Royal)	½ cup	18.9
(Jell-O)	½ cup	18.2
Dietetic (D-Zerta)	½ cup	Tr.
GELATIN DRINK (Knox)	1 envelope	14.0
GEL CUP (Del Monte):		
Lemon-lime with pineapple	5-oz. container	28.5
Orange with peaches	5-oz. container	26.5
Strawberry with peaches	5-oz. container	27.4
GERMAN DINNER (Swanson)	11-oz. dinner	42.2
GIN, SLOE (Garnier) 60 proof	1 fl. oz.	8.5
GINGER ALE, soft drink:		
Sweetened:		
(Canada Dry)	6 fl. oz.	16.2
(Clicquot Club) (Cott) (Dr. Brown's) (Key Food) (Mission) (Nedick's) (Waldbaum)	6 fl. oz.	15.0
(Yukon Club) golden	6 fl. oz.	16.1
(Schweppes)	6 fl. oz.	16.3
Low calorie:		
(Canada Dry)	6 fl. oz.	<1.0

*Prepared as Package Directs

Food and Description	Measure or Quantity	Carbohydrates (grams)
(Clicquot Club) (Cott) (Mission) (No-Cal) (Shasta)	6 fl. oz.	<.1
(Dr. Brown's) (Hoffman) (Key Food) (Waldbaum)	6 fl. oz.	.2
*GINGERBREAD MIX (Dromedary)	2″ x 2″ piece	18.8
GINGER, CANDIED	1 oz.	24.7
GOOSE	any quantity	0.
GOOSEBERRY	1 lb.	44.0
GOULASH DINNER (Chef Boy-Ar-Dee)	7⅓-oz. pkg.	32.4
GRANOLA:		
Sun Country, regular or almond	½ cup	34.0
Vita-Crunch:		
Regular	½ cup	45.1
Date	½ cup	47.0
Raisin	½ cup	46.4
Toasted almonds	½ cup	45.4
GRAPE:		
American type (slipskin)	1 lb.	44.8
European type (adherent skin)	1 lb.	69.8
GRAPEADE, chilled (Sealtest)	6 fl. oz.	24.2
GRAPE DRINK (Hi-C)	6 fl. oz.	21.8
*GRAPE DRINK MIX (Wyler's)	6 fl. oz.	15.4
GRAPE JELLY, low calorie (Kraft)	1 oz.	8.4
GRAPE JUICE:		
(Heinz)	5½ fl. oz.	31.3
*Frozen (Seneca)	½ cup	17.2
GRAPE-NUTS (Post)	1 oz.	23.0
GRAPE NUTS FLAKES (Post)	1 oz.	22.0

*Prepared as Package Directs

Food and Description	Measure or Quantity	Carbohydrates (grams)
GRAPE SOFT DRINK:		
Sweetened:		
(Canada Dry)	6 fl. oz.	23.9
(Dr. Brown's) (Key Food)		
(Waldbaum)	6 fl. oz.	21.9
(Fanta)	6 fl. oz.	23.9
Grapette	6 fl. oz.	23.4
(Hoffman) (Nedick's) (Yukon		
Club)	6 fl. oz.	23.2
(Nehi)	6 fl. oz.	22.3
(Salute)	6 fl. oz.	25.8
(Shasta)	6 fl. oz.	22.2
(Yoo-Hoo)	6 fl. oz.	18.0
High-protein (Yoo-Hoo)	6 fl. oz.	24.6
Low calorie:		
(Dr. Brown's) (Hoffman) (Key		
Food) (Waldbaum)	6 fl. oz.	.4
(No-Cal)	6 fl. oz.	0.
(Shasta) (Yukon Club)	6 fl. oz.	.1
GRAPEFRUIT:		
Pink & red:		
Seeded type	1 lb.	22.6
Seedless type	1 lb.	24.1
White:		
Seeded type	1 lb.	22.0
Seedless type	1 lb.	22.4
Bottled, chilled (Kraft):		
Sweetened, sections	4 oz.	12.5
Unsweetened, sections	4 oz.	10.4
Canned:		
(Stokely Van-Camp)	½ cup	20.4
Unsweetened (Del Monte)		
(Tillie Lewis)	½ cup	10.4
GRAPEFRUIT JUICE:		
Chilled, sweetened (Kraft)	½ cup	14.0
Canned:		
Sweetened (Heinz)	5½-fl.-oz. can	16.1
Unsweetened (Heinz)	5½-fl.-oz. can	11.8
Frozen:		
*Sweetened (Minute Maid)		
(Snow Crop)	½ cup	14.9

*Prepared as Package Directs

Food and Description	Measure or Quantity	Carbohydrates (grams)
*Unsweetened (Minute Maid) (Snow Crop)	½ cup	12.2
GRAPEFRUIT PEEL (Liberty)	1 oz.	22.6
GRAVY:		
Brown with onion (Franco-American)	1 cup	9.6
Ready Gravy	1 cup	29.6
GRAVY MASTER	1 fl. oz.	8.5
GRAVY with MEAT:		
Sliced beef (Bunker Hill)	15-oz. can	16.0
Frozen:		
Giblet & sliced turkey (Banquet)	2-lb. pkg.	22.0
Sliced beef (Morton House)	6¼ oz.	7.7
GRAVY MIX:		
Au jus (French's)	¾-oz. pkg.	8.7
Beef (Swiss Products)	1¼-oz. pkg.	22.6
Brown:		
(Durkee)	.8-oz. pkg.	10.5
(Lawry's)	1¼-oz. pkg.	16.3
(McCormick)	⅞-oz. pkg.	10.0
Chicken:		
(French's)	1¼-oz. pkg.	14.7
(Swiss)	⅞-oz. pkg.	15.9
Mushroom (Lawry's)	1.3-oz. pkg.	15.6
Onion (Durkee)	1-oz. pkg.	14.7
GRENADINE SYRUP (Giroux) non-alcoholic	1 fl. oz.	25.0
GUINEA HEN	any quantity	0.

H

Food and Description	Measure or Quantity	Carbohydrates (grams)
HADDOCK, raw or smoked	any quantity	0.
HADDOCK DINNER:		
(Banquet)	8.8-oz. dinner	44.8
(Weight Watchers)	18-oz. dinner	17.3
HALIBUT	any quantity	0.

*Prepared as Package Directs

Food and Description	Measure or Quantity	Carbohydrates (grams)
HAM:		
Boiled (Hormel)	1 oz.	0.
Canned:		
(Hormel)	1-lb. 8-oz. can	4.8
(Oscar Mayer) *Jubilee*, boneless	1 lb.	4.5
Chopped or minced (Armour Star)	1 oz.	.4
Chopped (Hormel)	1 oz.	.4
Deviled (Underwood)	4½-oz. can	Tr.
HAM & CHEESE LOAF (Oscar Mayer)	1-oz. slice	.3
HAM DINNER:		
(Banquet)	10-oz. dinner	53.2
(Morton)	10-oz. dinner	49.1
(Swanson)	10¼-oz. dinner	42.1
HAWAIIAN DINNER MIX (Hunt's) *Skillet*	1-lb. pkg.	122.3
HAWAIIAN PUNCH (RJR Foods)	6 fl. oz.	21.3
HAWAIIAN-STYLE VEGETABLES (Birds Eye)	10-oz. pkg.	37.8
HEADCHEESE (Oscar Mayer)	1-oz. slice	1.4
HERRING:		
Raw or kippered	any quantity	0.
Canned:		
Bismarck, drained (Vita)	5-oz. jar	6.9
In cream sauce (Vita)	8-oz. jar	18.1
HICKORY NUT, whole	1 lb.	20.3
HO-HO (Hostess) 10 to pkg.	1 piece	15.1
HOMINY GRITS (Quaker)	.8-oz. packet	17.6
HONEY	½ cup	134.1
HONEYDEW, whole	1 lb.	22.0

*Prepared as Package Directs

Food and Description	Measure or Quantity	Carbohydrates (grams)
HORSERADISH:		
Raw, whole	1 lb.	65.2
Prepared, cream style (Kraft)	1 oz.	.7

I

Food and Description	Measure or Quantity	Carbohydrates (grams)
ICE CREAM and FROZEN CUSTARD:		
10% fat	1 pt.	55.4
12% fat	1 pt.	58.6
16% fat	1 pt.	53.2
ICE CREAM BAR (Sealtest)	2½-fl.-oz. bar	12.1
ICE CREAM CONE, cone only:		
Assorted colors (Comet)	1 piece	3.9
Rolled sugar (Comet)	1 piece	10.2
ICE CREAM CUP, cup only:		
(Comet)	1 piece	4.1
Pilot (Comet)	1 piece	3.9
ICE CREAM SANDWICH (Sealtest)	3 fl. oz.	26.1
ICE MILK:		
(Borden) 3.5% fat	1 pt.	72.4
(Borden) *Lite-line*	1 pt.	64.0
Light n' Lively (Sealtest):		
Chocolate	1 pt.	76.8
Coffee	1 pt.	73.6
Strawberry	1 pt.	74.8
Vanilla	1 pt.	73.2
ICE CREAM BAR, chocolate-coated (Sealtest)	2½-fl.-oz. bar	13.6
ICE STICK (Sealtest)	3 fl. oz.	17.9
INDIAN PUDDING (B & M)	½ cup	27.1
ITALIAN DINNER:		
(Banquet)	11-oz. dinner	44.0
(Swanson)	13-oz. dinner	54.1

*Prepared as Package Directs

Food and Description	Measure or Quantity	Carbohydrates (grams)
ITALIAN-STYLE VEGETABLES (Birds Eye)	10-oz. pkg.	23.7

J

JACK MACKEREL, meat only	any quantity	0.
JAM	1 oz.	19.8
JAPANESE-STYLE VEGETA-BLES (Birds Eye)	10-oz. pkg.	17.4
JELLY (Kraft)	1 oz.	18.4
JERUSALEM ARTICHOKE, whole	1 lb.	52.3

K

KABOOM (General Mills)	1 oz.	24.6
KALE:		
Leaves including stems	1 lb.	20.1
Frozen, chopped (Birds Eye)	½ cup	4.2
KARO, syrup:		
Dark corn	1 cup	243.0
Light corn	1 cup	242.0
Pancake & waffle	1 cup	241.3
KIDNEY, beef	1 lb.	4.0
KING VITAMAN (Quaker)	1 oz.	24.0
KIRSCH LIQUEUR (Garnier) 96 proof	1 fl. oz.	8.8
KIX, cereal	1 oz.	23.8
KNOCKWURST (Oscar Mayer) *Chubbies*	2.4-oz. link	2.2
KOHLRABI, whole	1 lb.	21.9
*KOOL-AID (General Foods)	1 cup	25.0

*Prepared as Package Directs

Food and Description	Measure or Quantity	Carbohydrates (grams)
KRUMBLES (Kellogg's)	1 oz.	23.8
KUMQUAT, whole	1 lb.	72.1

L

Food and Description	Measure or Quantity	Carbohydrates (grams)
LAKE HERRING, raw	any quantity	0.
LAMB, raw	any quantity	0.
LAMB STEW, canned (B & M)	1 cup	11.4
LARD	any quantity	0.
LASAGNE:		
(Chef Boy-Ar-Dee)	40-oz. can	148.5
(Buitoni)	56-oz. pkg.	203.4
(Hunt's) *Skillet*	1-lb. 2-oz. pkg.	114.6
LEEKS, whole	1 lb.	26.4
LEMON, whole	1 lb.	48.1
LEMONADE:		
Chilled (Sealtest)	½ cup	13.4
Frozen, sweetened (ReaLemon)	6-oz. can	108.0
*LEMON CAKE MIX, pudding cake (Betty Crocker)	1 cake	272.4
LEMON JUICE:		
(Sunkist)	1 lemon	4.0
Canned, plastic container (ReaLemon)	1 T.	.8
Full strength, already reconstituted (Minute Maid) (Snow Crop)	½ cup	8.8
LEMON-LIME SOFT DRINK:		
Sweetened:		
(Dr. Brown's) (Hoffman) (Key Food) (Nedick's) (Shasta) (Waldbaum)	6 fl. oz.	18.4
(Salute)	6 fl. oz.	18.0

*Prepared as Package Directs

Food and Description	Measure or Quantity	Carbohydrates (grams)
Low calorie:		
(Hoffman)	6 fl. oz.	.2
(Shasta)	6 fl. oz.	<.1
(Yukon Club)	6 fl. oz.	.4
LEMON PEEL, candied (Liberty)	1 oz.	22.6
LEMON PIE, cream, frozen:		
(Morton)	14.4-oz. pie	145.6
(Mrs. Smith's)	8″ pie	190.0
LEMON PIE FILLING:		
(Comstock)	½ cup	44.0
(Lucky Leaf)	8 oz.	95.4
LEMON PUDDING (Hunt's)	5-oz. can	35.3
LEMON PUDDING or PIE MIX:		
*(Royal) including crust	9″ pie	318.4
*Instant (Jell-O)	½ cup	30.5
LEMON SOFT DRINK:		
Sweetened:		
(Canada Dry) *Hi-Spot*	6 fl. oz.	18.4
(Clicquot Club) (Cott) (Mission)	6 fl. oz.	18.0
(Royal Crown)	6 fl. oz.	22.2
Low calorie:		
(Canada Dry)	6 fl. oz.	<1.0
(Clicquot Club) (Cott) (Mission)	6 fl. oz.	.5
(No-Cal)	6 fl. oz.	0.
LENTIL:		
Whole, dry	½ lb.	136.3
Split, dry	½ lb.	140.2
LENTIL SOUP, with ham (Crosse & Blackwell)	13-oz. can	34.0
LETTUCE:		
Bibb, Boston	1 lb.	8.4
Grand Rapids, Romaine, Simpson	1 lb.	10.2
Iceberg, New York	1 lb.	12.5
LIEBFRAUMILCH WINE (Julius Kayser) Glockenspiel, 10% alcohol	3 fl. oz.	1.8

*Prepared as Package Directs

Food and Description	Measure or Quantity	Carbohydrates (grams)
LIFE, cereal	1 oz.	20.2
LIKE, soft drink	6 fl. oz.	.3
LIME	1 lime	4.9
LIMEADE (ReaLemon)	6-oz. can	108.0
LIME JUICE, plastic container, *ReaLime*	1 T.	.5
LIME PIE (Banquet)	2½-oz. serving	27.5
LITCHI NUT, dried, whole	¼ lb.	36.9
LIVER, raw:		
Beef	1 lb.	24.0
Calf	1 lb.	18.6
Chicken	1 lb.	13.2
Hog	1 lb.	11.8
Lamb	1 lb.	13.2
LIVERWURST (Oscar Mayer)	.9-oz. slice	.4
LIVERWURST SPREAD (Underwood)	1 T.	.5
LOBSTER, whole	1 lb.	.6
LOBSTER NEWBURG (Stouffer's)	11½-oz. pkg.	16.0
LOBSTER SOUP (Crosse & Blackwell)	13-oz. can	13.0
LOG CABIN, syrup	1 T.	12.2
LUNCHEON MEAT:		
All meat (Oscar Mayer)	1-oz. slice	.9
Cocktail loaf (Oscar Mayer)	1-oz. slice	3.8
Luxury Loaf (Oscar Mayer)	1-oz. slice	1.3
Olive loaf (Oscar Mayer)	1-oz. slice	2.6
Pickle & pimento (Sugardale)	1-oz. slice	Tr.
Spiced (Hormel)	1 oz.	<1.0

*Prepared as Package Directs

M

Food and Description	Measure or Quantity	Carbohydrates (grams)
MACADAMIA NUT, shelled	4 oz.	18.0
MACARONI:		
Dry	1 oz.	21.3
20% Protein (Buitoni)	1 oz.	18.2
MACARONI & BEEF:		
Canned, tiny meatballs & sauce (Buitoni)	4 oz.	12.3
Frozen:		
(Banquet)	2-lb. pkg.	101.5
With tomatoes (Stouffer's)	11½-oz. pkg.	39.0
MACARONI & CHEESE:		
(Heinz)	8¼-oz. can	27.0
Frozen:		
(Banquet)	20-oz. pkg.	82.0
(Morton)	8-oz. casserole	31.5
MACARONI DINNER:		
& cheese:		
*(Chef Boy-Ar-Dee)	4½-oz. pkg.	33.8
(Banquet)	12-oz. dinner	47.0
Creole, with mushrooms (Heinz)	8¾-oz. can	28.4
MACARONI SALAD, canned (Nalley's)	4 oz.	13.9
MACKEREL	any quantity	0.
MADEIRA WINE (Leacock) 19% alcohol	3 fl. oz.	6.3
MAI TAI COCKTAIL:		
(Lemon Hart) 48 proof	3 fl. oz.	15.6
(National Distillers) *Duet*, 12% alcohol	8-fl.-oz. can	28.8
(Party Tyme) 12½% alcohol	2 fl. oz.	5.7
Dry mix (Bar-Tender's)	1 serving	17.0
Dry mix (Party Tyme)	1 serving	11.8
Liquid mix (Party Tyme)	2 fl. oz.	11.2
MALTEX, cereal	1 oz.	22.7

*Prepared as Package Directs

Food and Description	Measure or Quantity	Carbohydrates (grams)
MALT LIQUOR, *Country Club*	12 fl. oz.	2.8
MANDARIN ORANGE, CANNED:		
(Del Monte)	½ cup	20.6
(Diet Delight)	½ cup	7.4
(S and W) *Nutradiet*	4 oz.	7.1
MANGO, whole	1 lb.	51.1
MANHATTAN COCKTAIL:		
(Hiram Walker) 55 proof	3 fl. oz.	3.0
(National Distillers) *Duet*, 20% alcohol	8-fl.-oz. can	11.2
(Party Tyme) 20% alcohol	2 fl. oz.	1.5
Brandy (National Distillers) *Duet*, 20% alcohol	8-fl.-oz. can	8.0
Dry mix (Bar-Tender's)	1 serving	5.6
MANICOTTI, with sauce (Buitoni)	4 oz.	16.1
MAPLE SYRUP (Cary's)	1 T.	15.7
***MARBLE CAKE MIX** (Betty Crocker)	1 cake	446.4
MARGARINE	1 lb.	1.8
MARGARINE, IMITATION (Mazola)	1 lb.	0.
MARGARINE, WHIPPED	1 cup	.6
MARGARITA COCKTAIL:		
(National Distillers) *Duet*, 12½% alcohol	8-fl.-oz. can	20.0
(Party Tyme) 12½% alcohol	2 fl. oz.	5.7
Dry mix (Bar-Tender's)	1 serving	17.3
Dry mix (Party Tyme)	½-oz. serving	11.5
Liquid mix (Party Tyme)	2 fl. oz.	14.9
MARINADE MIX:		
(Adolph's)	.8-oz. pkg.	8.5
(Durkee)	.9-oz. pkg.	9.9
(Lawry's)	1.6-oz. pkg.	15.1

*Prepared as Package Directs

Food and Description	Measure or Quantity	Carbohydrates (grams)
MARMALADE:		
Sweetened (Kraft)	1 oz.	19.3
Low calorie (Kraft)	1 oz.	8.6
MARTINI COCKTAIL		
Gin:		
(Hiram Walker) 67.5 proof	3 fl. oz.	.6
(National Distillers) *Duet*, 21% alcohol	8-fl.-oz. can	1.6
(Party Tyme) 24% alcohol	2 fl. oz.	0.
Liquid mix (Party Tyme)	2 fl. oz.	3.2
Vodka:		
(Hiram Walker) 60 proof	3 fl. oz.	0.
(National Distillers) *Duet*, 20% alcohol	8-fl.-oz. can	1.6
(Party Tyme) 21% alcohol	2 fl. oz.	0.
***MASA HARINA** (Quaker)	2 tortillas	27.9
***MASO TRIGO** (Quaker)	2 tortillas	24.6
MATZO:		
Regular (Manischewitz)	1 matzo	28.1
Tea (Goodman's)	1 matzo	12.9
Unsalted (Horowitz-Margareten)	1 matzo	28.2
MATZO MEAL (Manischewitz)	1 cup	96.2
MAYONNAISE:		
(Best Foods) *Real;* (Hellmann's)	1 T.	<.1
(Kraft)	1 T.	.1
Saffola	1 T.	2.9
MAYPO, cereal	1 oz.	19.8
MEATBALL:		
In sauce (Prince)	3.7-oz. can	8.1
With gravy (Chef Boy-Ar-Dee)	15¼-oz. can	18.4
MEAT LOAF ENTREE (Swanson)	9-oz. pkg.	20.2
MEAT LOAF DINNER:		
(Banquet)	11-oz. dinner	28.8

*Prepared as Package Directs

Food and Description	Measure or Quantity	Carbohydrates (grams)
(Morton) 3-course	1-lb. 1-oz. dinner	69.4
(Swanson) 3-course	16-oz. dinner	52.8
MEAT LOAF SEASONING MIX		
(Contadina)	3¾-oz. pkg.	70.1
MEAT, POTTED:		
(Armour Star)	3-oz. can	0.
(Hormel)	3-oz. can	1.0
MELBA TOAST:		
Garlic, onion, plain or sesame (Keebler)	1 piece	1.5
Garlic or onion rounds (Old London)	1 piece	1.4
Pumpernickel, rye, wheat or white (Old London)	1 piece	3.1
MELON BALL, in syrup	½ cup	18.2
MEXICAN DINNER:		
Mix (Hunt's) *Skillet*	1-lb. 2-oz. pkg.	130.0
Frozen:		
Mexican style (Banquet)	16¼-oz. dinner	74.0
(Swanson)	18-oz. dinner	71.3
MEXICAN-STYLE VEGETA-BLES (Birds Eye)	10-oz. pkg.	51.0
MILK,CONDENSED, *Eagle Brand*	1 fl. oz.	21.1
MILK, DRY, nonfat, instant (Carnation)	1 cup	37.4
MILK, EVAPORATED (Borden)	14.5-oz. can	39.9
MILK, FRESH:		
Whole, 3.5% fat (Sealtest)	1 cup	11.0
Skim:		
Light n' Lively (Sealtest)	1 cup	13.6
Skim-line (Borden)	1 cup	13.6
Buttermilk:		
1% fat (Borden)	1 cup	12.4
Light n' Lively (Sealtest)	1 cup	10.5

*Prepared as Package Directs

Food and Description	Measure or Quantity	Carbohydrates (grams)
Chocolate milk drink, fresh:		
With whole milk 3.3% fat		
(Meadow Gold)	1 cup	37.0
With skim milk, 1% fat (Sealtest)	1 cup	26.2
MINCEMEAT:		
(Crosse & Blackwell)	1 cup	228.8
Condensed (None Such)	9-oz. pkg.	221.2
MINCE PIE:		
(Morton)	20-oz. pie	214.8
(Mrs. Smith's)	8″ pie	310.0
MINESTRONE SOUP (Campbell)	1 can	21.0
MOLASSES:		
Dark (Brer Rabbit)	1 T.	13.3
Light (Brer Rabbit)	1 T.	14.6
Unsulphured (Grandma's)	1 T.	13.7
MORTADELLA	1 oz.	.2
MRS. BUTTERWORTH'S SYRUP	1 T.	13.0
MUFFIN:		
Blueberry, frozen (Morton)	1.6-oz. muffin	20.8
Bran (Thomas') with raisins	1.9-oz. muffin	26.7
Corn (Thomas')	2-oz. muffin	26.8
English (Thomas')	2.1-oz. muffin	28.4
Scone (Wonder) *Raisin Round*	1 piece	30.2
MUFFIN MIX:		
*Blueberry (Betty Crocker)	2¾″ muffin	19.3
*Corn (Flako)	1.3-oz. muffin	20.4
*Honey bran (Betty Crocker)	2¾″ muffin	26.2
MUSHROOM:		
Raw, whole	½ lb.	9.7
Canned:		
(Oxford Royal)	4-oz. can	2.4
Sliced (B in B)	6-oz. can	4.1
Frozen, in butter sauce		
(Green Giant)	6-oz. pkg.	6.0

*Prepared as Package Directs

Food and Description	Measure or Quantity	Carbohydrates (grams)
MUSHROOM SOUP, cream of (Heinz) *Great American*	1 cup	12.4
MUSHROOM SOUP MIX, cream of (Lipton) *Cup-a-Soup*	1 pkg.	9.6
MUSSEL, Atlantic & Pacific	1 lb.	7.2
MUSTARD:		
Brown (French's) (Gulden's)	1 tsp.	.5
Grey Poupon	1 tsp.	.4
Yellow (Gulden's) (Heinz)	1 tsp.	.5
MUSTARD GREENS:		
Raw, whole	1 lb.	17.8
Chopped (Birds Eye)	½ cup	2.2

N

Food and Description	Measure or Quantity	Carbohydrates (grams)
NEAPOLITAN CREAM PIE:		
(Morton)	14.4-oz. pie	141.6
(Mrs. Smith's)	8″ pie	200.0
NECTARINE, whole	1 lb.	71.4
NOODLE, dry, 1½″ strips	1 oz.	20.4
NOODLE & BEEF:		
(Heinz)	8½-oz. can	18.1
(Nalley's)	2-lb. pkg.	102.0
NOODLE, CHOW MEIN (Hung's)	1 oz.	16.1
*****NOODLE DINNER,** Stroganoff mix (Betty Crocker)	1 cup	41.6
NOODLE MIX:		
*Almondine (Betty Crocker)	½ cup	26.2
*Romanoff, *Noodle-Roni*	4 oz.	22.5
NUT, mixed:		
Dry roasted:		
(Flavor House)	1 oz.	5.4
(Skippy)	1 oz.	5.7

*Prepared as Package Directs

Food and Description	Measure or Quantity	Carbohydrates (grams)
Oil roasted:		
With peanuts (Planters)	1 oz.	6.2
Without peanuts (Planters)	1 oz.	6.0

O

Food and Description	Measure or Quantity	Carbohydrates (grams)
OAT FLAKES (Post)	1 oz.	19.0
OATMEAL:		
Instant (Quaker)	1-oz. packet	19.0
Quick (H-O)	1 cup	45.8
Regular:		
(Ralston)	1 oz.	20.3
*(Albers) old fashioned	1 cup	26.0
OCEAN PERCH, raw	any quantity	0.
OCEAN PERCH MEALS, frozen:		
(Banquet)	8.8-oz. dinner	49.2
(Weight Watchers)	18-oz. dinner	18.4
OIL, salad or cooking	any quantity	0.
OKRA:		
Raw, whole	1 lb.	29.6
Cut (Birds Eye)	½ cup	7.6
Whole (Birds Eye)	½ cup	5.7
OLD FASHIONED:		
Cocktail (Hiram Walker) 62 proof	3 fl. oz.	3.0
Mix (Bar-Tender's)	1 serving	4.7
OLIVE:		
Greek style, pitted	1 oz.	2.5
Green, pitted & drained	1 oz.	.4
Ripe	1 oz.	.7
ONION:		
Raw, whole	1 lb.	35.9
Canned (Comstock-Greenwood)	4 oz.	7.4
Dehydrated, flakes	½ cup	26.2
Frozen:		
Chopped (Birds Eye)	¼ cup	2.5
Whole, small (Birds Eye)	½ cup	12.0

*Prepared as Package Directs

Food and Description	Measure or Quantity	Carbohydrates (grams)
Small with cream sauce (Birds Eye)	9-oz. pkg.	38.1
French-fried rings:		
(Durkee) *O & C*	3-oz. can	30.8
(Mrs. Paul's)	9-oz. pkg.	50.5
Pickled, cocktail (Crosse & Blackwell)	1 T.	.3
ONION, GREEN, raw, whole	1 lb.	35.7
ONION SOUP (Hormel)	15-oz. can	5.5
ONION SOUP MIX (Lipton)		
Cup-a-Soup	1 pkg.	5.4
ONION, WELSH, raw, whole	1 lb.	19.2
ORANGE:		
California Navel	1 lb.	39.2
California Valencia	1 lb.	42.2
Florida	1 lb.	40.3
ORANGEADE, chilled (Sealtest)	½ cup	15.6
ORANGE CAKE, frosted (Sara Lee)	2 oz.	30.0
ORANGE CREAM BAR (Sealtest)	2½-fl.-oz. bar	17.6
ORANGE DRINK (Hi-C)	6 fl. oz.	22.2
***ORANGE-GRAPEFRUIT JUICE**		
(Minute Maid) (Snow Crop)	½ cup	12.7
ORANGE ICE (Sealtest)	1 pt.	130.4
ORANGE JUICE:		
Fresh	½ cup	12.9
Chilled (Kraft)	½ cup	13.8
Canned, sweetened (Heinz)	5½-fl.-oz. can	21.0
Canned, unsweetened (Heinz)	5½-fl.-oz. can	16.5
Frozen:		
*(Lake Hamilton) (Nature's Best)	½ cup	13.3
*(Minute Maid) (Snow Crop)	½ cup	13.7

*Prepared as Package Directs

Food and Description	Measure or Quantity	Carbohydrates (grams)
ORANGE PEEL, candied (Liberty)	1 oz.	22.6
***ORANGE PLUS** (Birds Eye)	½ cup	16.6
ORANGE SOFT DRINK:		
Sweetened:		
(Canada Dry) *Sunripe*	6 fl. oz.	24.6
(Clicquot Club) (Cott) (Mission)	6 fl. oz.	25.0
(Dr. Brown's) (Nedick's)		
(Waldbaum)	6 fl. oz.	22.6
(Fanta) (Yukon Club)	6 fl. oz.	23.8
(Hoffman)	6 fl. oz.	23.2
(Key Food)	6 fl. oz.	21.5
(Kirsch)	6 fl. oz.	21.9
(Nehi)	6 fl. oz.	24.8
(Salute)	6 fl. oz.	25.2
(Shasta)	6 fl. oz.	24.0
(Yoo-Hoo)	6 fl. oz.	18.0
High-protein (Yoo-Hoo)	6 fl. oz.	24.6
Low calorie:		
(Canada Dry) (Shasta)	6 fl. oz.	<.1
(Clicquot Club) (Cott) (Mission)	6 fl. oz.	.3
(Dr. Brown's) (Hoffman) (Key		
Food) (Waldbaum)	6 fl. oz.	.2
(Nedick's) (Yukon Club)	6 fl. oz.	.4
(No-Cal)	6 fl. oz.	0.
ORIENTAL DINNER (Hunt's)		
Skillet	1-lb. 1-oz. pkg.	119.3
OVALTINE, dry	1 oz.	24.0
OYSTER:		
Eastern, in shell	1 lb.	1.5
Eastern, meat only	1 lb.	15.6
Pacific & Western, meat only	1 lb.	29.2
OYSTER STEW (Campbell)	1 can	23.2

P

PANCAKE (Swanson)	6-oz. breakfast	41.6
PANCAKE & WAFFLE MIX:		
*Buckwheat (Aunt Jemima)	4″ pancake	8.0
Buttermilk (Pillsbury) *Hungry Jack*	1 oz.	20.5

*Prepared as Package Directs

Food and Description	Measure or Quantity	Carbohydrates (grams)
Plain:		
*(Aunt Jemima) Complete	4" pancake	11.4
*(Aunt Jemima) Easy Pour	4" pancake	10.9
*(Aunt Jemima) Original	4" pancake	7.8
PARISIAN-STYLE VEGETA-		
BLES (Birds Eye)	10-oz. pkg.	22.2
PARSLEY, fresh, whole	½ lb.	19.3
PARSNIP, raw, whole	1 lb.	67.5
PASSION FRUIT, whole	1 lb.	50.0
PASTINAS, dry, egg	1 oz.	20.4
PASTRAMI (Vienna)	1 oz.	.4
PASTRY SHELL:		
Pot pie, bland (Keebler)	4" shell	29.6
Frozen, tart (Pepperidge Farm)	3-oz. pie tart	32.8
PATE:		
Liver (Hormel)	1 oz.	1.1
Liver (Sell's)	1 oz.	1.0
PEA, GREEN:		
Raw, in pod	1 lb.	24.8
Raw, shelled	1 lb.	65.3
Canned:		
Early (Le Sueur)	8.5-oz. can	22.0
Sweet (Green Giant)	8.5-oz. can	21.2
Frozen:		
(Birds Eye)	10-oz. pkg.	36.6
In butter sauce (Green Giant)		
Le Sueur	10-oz. pkg.	33.0
With cream sauce (Green Giant)	10-oz. pkg.	32.1
With sliced mushroom (Birds Eye)	10-oz. pkg.	35.1
PEA, MATURE SEED, raw:		
Whole	1 lb.	273.5
Split (Sinsheimer)	1 lb.	280.0

*Prepared as Package Directs

Food and Description	Measure or Quantity	Carbohydrates (grams)
PEA POD, raw, whole	1 lb.	51.7
PEA & CARROT:		
(Del Monte)	½ cup	8.9
Frozen:		
(Birds Eye)	10-oz. pkg.	26.1
In cream sauce (Green Giant)	10-oz. pkg.	29.1
PEA & CELERY (Birds Eye)	10-oz. pkg.	29.4
PEA & ONION, in butter sauce (Green Giant)	10-oz. pkg.	29.1
PEA & POTATO (Birds Eye)	1 pkg.	44.7
PEA SOUP, GREEN:		
Canned (Campbell)	1 can	42.0
Dry mix (Lipton) *Cup-a-Soup*	1.2-oz. pkg.	22.1
PEA SOUP, SPLIT:		
(Manischewitz)	1 can	45.2
With smoked ham (Heinz) *Great American*	1 cup	24.0
PEACH:		
Fresh	1 lb.	38.3
Canned:		
Heavy syrup (Hunt's)	½ cup	25.7
Spiced (Del Monte)	½ cup	29.9
Canned, dietetic:		
(Blue Boy)	4 oz.	7.4
(Diet Delight) freestone	½ cup	15.1
(Tillie Lewis) Elberta	½ cup	9.4
Dried (Del Monte)	½ cup	51.0
Frozen (Birds Eye)	½ cup	22.3
PEACH NECTAR (Del Monte)	1 cup	37.9
PEACH PIE:		
(Morton)	20-oz. pie	209.4
(Mrs. Smith's)	8" pie	250.0
PEACH PIE FILLING:		
(Comstock)	½ cup	47.1
(Lucky Leaf)	8 oz.	74.0

*Prepared as Package Directs

Food and Description	Measure or Quantity	Carbohydrates (grams)
PEACH TURNOVER (Pepperidge Farm)	1 turnover	33.4
PEANUT:		
In shell	1 lb.	61.6
Roasted:		
Dry (Franklin)	1 oz.	5.4
Dry (Skippy)	1 oz.	4.4
Oil (Planters) cocktail	1 oz.	5.0
Spanish, dry roasted (Planters)	1 oz.	3.4
Spanish, oil roasted (Planters)	1 oz.	3.4
PEANUT BUTTER:		
(Bama) crunchy	1 T.	3.3
(Bama) smooth	1 T.	3.6
(Peter Pan)	1 T.	3.9
(Skippy)	1 T.	2.2
PEANUT SPREAD, diet (Peter Pan)	1 T.	2.0
PEAR:		
Fresh, whole	1 lb.	63.2
Canned:		
Juice pack (Libby's)	4 oz.	17.8
Heavy syrup (Hunt's)	½ cup	23.9
Unsweetened (S and W) *Nutradiet*	2 halves	7.7
Dried (Del Monte)	½ cup	46.4
PEAR NECTAR (Del Monte)	1 cup	38.4
PECAN:		
In shell	1 lb.	35.1
Shelled	1 lb.	66.2
Dry, roasted (Planters)	1 oz.	3.5
PECAN PIE:		
(Morton)	20-oz. pie	296.4
(Mrs. Smith's)	8″ pie	350.0
PEPPER:		
Black	1 tsp.	.7
Seasoned (Lawry's)	1.6-oz. pkg.	29.8
PEPPER, HOT CHILI:		
Green, raw	4 oz.	7.5

*Prepared as Package Directs

Food and Description	Measure or Quantity	Carbohydrates (grams)
Red:		
Raw	4 oz.	20.5
Canned, drained (Ortega)	¼ cup	1.9
Dried (Chili Products)	1 oz.	16.9
PEPPER, STUFFED, with veal		
(Weight Watchers)	12-oz. dinner	13.6
PEPPER, SWEET, raw:		
Green, whole	1 lb.	17.9
Red, whole	1 lb.	25.8
PERCH:		
Raw	any quantity	0.
Frozen, breaded (Gorton)	11-oz. pkg.	27.0
PERNOD (Julius Wile) 90 proof	1 fl. oz.	1.1
PERSIMMON, Japanese or Kaki:		
With seeds	1 lb.	73.3
Seedless	1 lb.	75.1
PHEASANT, ready-to-cook	any quantity	0.
PICKLE:		
Cucumber, fresh or bread &		
butter (Aunt Jane's)	4 slices or sticks	5.1
Dill, *L & S*	1 large pickle	2.0
Dill, candied (Smucker's)	4" pickle	11.2
Kosher dill (Smucker's)	3½" pickle	1.4
Sour (Heinz)	2" pickle	.2
Sweet:		
Gherkin (Bond's)	1 pickle	3.0
Mixed (Heinz)	3 pieces	5.6
PIECRUST:		
(Mrs. Smith's)	8" shell	48.0
(Mrs. Smith's) old fashioned	9" shell	75.0
(Mrs. Smith's)	10" shell	100.0
PIECRUST MIX:		
*Graham cracker (Betty Crocker)	1 crust	133.8
*(Flako)	9" shell	72.0

*Prepared as Package Directs

Food and Description	Measure or Quantity	Carbohydrates (grams)
PIGS FEET, pickled (Hormel)	1-pt. can	.2
PIKE, raw	any quantity	0.
PILLSBURY INSTANT BREAKFAST	1 oz.	19.0
PIMIENTO (Ortega)	¼ cup	1.3
PINA COLADA MIX (Party Tyme)	½-oz. pkg.	13.2
PINCH of HERBS (Lawry's)	2.2-oz. pkg.	21.9
PINEAPPLE:		
Fresh, whole	1 lb.	32.3
Canned:		
Juice pack:		
Chunks or crushed (Dole)	½ cup (includes 2½ T. juice)	15.5
Slices (Dole)	2 med. slices & 2½ T. juice	21.7
Heavy syrup (Del Monte)	½ cup	26.8
Unsweetened (S and W) *Nutradiet*	2½ slices	13.1
PINEAPPLE, CANDIED (Liberty)	1 oz.	22.6
PINEAPPLE & GRAPEFRUIT JUICE DRINK (Dole) regular or pink	6-fl.-oz. can	25.2
PINEAPPLE JUICE:		
(Heinz)	5½-fl.-oz. can	23.5
(Dole)	6-fl.-oz. can	26.0
PINEAPPLE PIE (Morton)	46-oz. pie	484.8
PINEAPPLE PIE FILLING:		
(Comstock)	½ cup	35.7
(Lucky Leaf)	8 oz.	59.0
PINE NUT:		
Pignolias, shelled	4 oz.	13.2
Piñon, shelled	4 oz.	23.2

*Prepared as Package Directs

Food and Description	Measure or Quantity	Carbohydrates (grams)
PISTACHIO NUT:		
In shell	4 oz.	10.8
Dry, roasted (Flavor House)	1 oz.	5.4
PIZZA PIE, frozen:		
With cheese (Chef Boy-Ar-Dee)	12½" pie	108.0
With cheese (Kraft)	14-oz. pie	98.9
With pepperoni (Chef Boy-Ar-Dee)	14-oz. pie	108.6
With sausage, *Pee Wee* (Kraft)	2½-oz. pie	19.7
PIZZA PIE MIX:		
*With cheese (Chef Boy-Ar-Dee)	15½-oz. pie	132.5
*With sausage (Chef Boy-Ar-Dee)	17-oz. pie	135.0
PIZZA SAUCE:		
(Chef Boy-Ar-Dee)	10¼-oz. can	11.0
Mix (French's)	1-oz. pkg.	17.2
PIZZARIA MIX (Hunt's) *Skillet*	14.1-oz. pkg.	80.9
PLANTAIN, whole	1 lb.	101.9
PLUM:		
Fresh, Japanese & hybrid	1 lb.	52.4
Fresh, prune-type	1 lb.	84.0
Canned, heavy syrup (Del Monte)	½ cup	30.4
Canned, unsweetened (Tillie Lewis)	½ cup	14.7
PLUM PUDDING (Crosse & Blackwell)	4 oz.	62.4
POLISH-STYLE SAUSAGE:		
(Oscar Mayer) all meat	1 oz.	.5
Kolbase (Hormel)	1 oz.	.4
POLYNESIAN-STYLE DINNER (Swanson)	11¾-oz. dinner	62.4
POMEGRANATE, whole	1 lb.	41.7
POMMARD WINE:		
(B & G) 13% alcohol	3 fl. oz.	.4
(Chanson) 11½% alcohol	3 fl. oz.	6.3

*Prepared as Package Directs

Food and Description	Measure or Quantity	Carbohydrates (grams)
POMPANO, whole, raw	any quantity	0.
POPCORN:		
(Jiffy Pop)	5-oz. pkg.	59.6
(Tom Houston)	1 cup	8.9
Buttered (Jiffy Pop)	5-oz. pkg.	58.8
Cracker Jack	1 cup	11.3
Cheese (Wise)	⅝-oz. bag	9.6
*POPOVER, mix (Flako)	1 pkg.	135.0
PORGY, whole, raw	any quantity	0.
PORK:		
Fresh, raw	any quantity	0.
Cured:		
Boston butt, raw	any quantity	0.
Ham:		
Raw	any quantity	0.
Fully cooked, bone-in (Hormel)	1 lb.	2.8
Fully cooked, boneless:		
Parti-Style (Armour Star)	1 lb.	.4
Festival, smoked (Wilson)	1 lb.	4.0
Picnic:		
Raw	any quantity	0.
Canned (Hormel)	3-lb. can	2.4
PORK DINNER (Swanson)	10-oz. dinner	40.5
PORK SAUSAGE:		
(Armour Star)	1-oz. sausage	0.
Little Friers (Oscar Mayer)	1-oz. link	.2
PORK, SWEET & SOUR (Chun King)	15-oz. pkg.	52.0
PORT WINE:		
(Gallo) 16% alcohol	3 fl. oz.	7.8
(Italian Swiss Colony-Gold Medal) 19.7% alcohol	3 fl. oz.	8.7
(Louis M. Martini) 19½% alcohol	3 fl. oz.	2.0
(Robertson's) tawny, 21% alcohol	3 fl. oz.	9.9

*Prepared as Package Directs

Food and Description	Measure or Quantity	Carbohydrates (grams)
POST TOASTIES (Post)	1 oz.	24.0
***POSTUM**	1 cup	3.7
POTATO:		
Raw, whole	1 lb.	62.8
Canned, white (Butter Kernel)	3-4 small potatoes	22.0
Frozen:		
Au gratin (Stouffer's)	11½-oz. pkg.	35.6
Stuffed, baked, with cheese (Holloway House)	1 potato	28.0
Stuffed, baked, with sour cream & chives (Holloway House)	1 potato	27.4
POTATO CHIP:		
(Pringle's)	10 chips	7.7
(Wise)	1-oz. bag	14.8
Barbecue (Wise)	1-oz. bag	15.0
Ridgies (Wise)	1-oz. bag	14.7
POTATO MIX:		
Au gratin (French's)	5½-oz. pkg.	92.0
Mashed, country style (French's)	2⅔-oz. pkg.	60.0
Scalloped (French's)	5⅝-oz. pkg.	117.0
Whipped (Borden)	1 cup	48.0
POTATO PANCAKE MIX (French's)	3-oz. pkg.	62.0
POTATO SALAD, canned (Nalley's)	4 oz.	20.2
POTATO STICK:		
(Durkee) *O & C*	1¾-oz. can	24.8
Julienne (Wise)	1-oz. bag	15.6
POUILLY-FUISSE WINE (B & G) 12½% alcohol	3 fl. oz.	.3
POUILLY-FUME (B & G) 12% alcohol	3 fl. oz.	.1
POUND CAKE:		
Plain (Drake's)	9-oz. cake	147.4
Plain (Sara Lee)	1 oz.	13.0

*Prepared as Package Directs

Food and Description	Measure or Quantity	Carbohydrates (grams)
PRESERVE (Kraft)	1 oz.	19.3
PRETZEL:		
(Nabisco) *Mister Salty*, Dutch	½-oz. piece	11.2
(Nabisco) *Mister Salty Veri-Thin* sticks	1 piece	.2
(Old London) nuggets	2-oz. bag	44.1
PRODUCT 19 (Kellogg's)	1 oz.	23.1
PRUNE:		
Dried (Del Monte)	½ cup	58.7
Canned (Sunsweet)	1 cup	72.0
PRUNE JUICE:		
(Bennett's)	½ cup	24.0
(Heinz)	5½-fl.-oz. can	28.3
PULIGNY MONTRACHET WINE		
(B & G) 12% alcohol	3 fl. oz.	.3
PUMPKIN:		
Fresh, whole	1 lb.	20.6
Canned (Libby's)	½ cup	10.3
PUMPKIN PIE:		
(Banquet)	5-oz. serving	46.5
(Morton)	20-oz. pie	157.2
(Mrs. Smith's)	8″ pie	201.6
PUMPKIN PIE FILLING		
(Comstock)	1 cup	90.2
PUMPKIN SEED, hulled	4 oz.	17.0

Q

Food and Description	Measure or Quantity	Carbohydrates (grams)
QUAKE, cereal	1 oz.	23.1
QUININE SOFT DRINK or TONIC WATER:		
Sweetened:		
(Canada Dry)	6 fl. oz.	17.6

*Prepared as Package Directs

Food and Description	Measure or Quantity	Carbohydrates (grams)
(Dr. Brown's) (Hoffman) (Schweppes)	6 fl. oz.	16.5
(Fanta)	6 fl. oz.	15.7
(Kirsch)	6 fl. oz.	11.8
(Shasta)	6 fl. oz.	14.4
(Yukon Club)	6 fl. oz.	16.7
Low calorie (No-Cal)	6 fl. oz.	0.

R

RABBIT, ready-to-cook	any quantity	0.
RADISH, raw, without tops	½ lb.	7.4
RAISIN:		
Seeded, Muscat (Sun-Maid)	15-oz. pkg.	302.8
Seedless, golden (Sun-Maid)	15-oz. pkg.	334.0
RASPBERRY:		
Fresh, black	½ lb.	34.6
Fresh, red	½ lb.	29.9
Frozen (Birds Eye)	½ cup	37.2
RASPBERRY SOFT DRINK:		
Sweetened:		
(Clicquot Club) (Cott) (Mission)	6 fl. oz.	24.0
(Dr. Brown's)	6 fl. oz.	21.5
(Hoffman) (Shasta) (Yukon Club)	6 fl. oz.	22.3
(Kirsch)	6 fl. oz.	22.1
Low calorie:		
(Clicquot Club) (Cott) (Dr. Brown's) (Hoffman) (Key Food) (Mission) (Waldbaum)	6 fl. oz.	.4
(No-Cal)	6 fl. oz.	<.1
(Shasta)	6 fl. oz.	.1
RASPBERRY TURNOVER (Pepperidge Farm)	1 turnover	3.0
RAVIOLI:		
Meat (Chef Boy-Ar-Dee)	40-oz. can	151.0
Cheese (Chef Boy-Ar-Dee)	15-oz. can	63.0
Frozen:		
Beef (Kraft)	12½-oz. pkg.	49.9

*Prepared as Package Directs

Food and Description	Measure or Quantity	Carbohydrates (grams)
Cheese (Kraft)	12½-oz. pkg.	48.1
RED & GRAY SNAPPER, whole	any quantity	0.
RELISH:		
Barbecue (Heinz)	1 T.	8.5
Corn (Crosse & Blackwell)	1 T.	3.6
Hamburger (Del Monte)	1 T.	8.9
Hot dog (Heinz)	1 T.	3.9
India (Crosse & Blackwell)	1 T.	6.3
Piccalilli (Heinz)	1 T.	5.3
Sweet (Lutz & Schramm)	1 T.	4.0
RHINE WINE:		
(Gallo) Rhine Garten, 12% alcohol	3 fl. oz.	3.0
(Italian Swiss Colony-Gold Medal) 11.6% alcohol	3 fl. oz.	.6
(Taylor) 12½% alcohol	3 fl. oz.	Tr.
RHUBARB:		
Raw, partly trimmed	1 lb.	12.6
Frozen (Birds Eye)	½ cup	21.4
RICE:		
Brown, raw	1 oz.	21.9
White, raw:		
Instant	1 oz.	23.4
Parboiled, long-grain	1 oz.	23.0
Regular	1 oz.	22.6
White & wild (Green Giant)	12-oz. pkg.	68.1
RICE CHEX (Ralston)	1 oz.	24.9
RICE, FRIED:		
Frozen:		
With almonds (Green Giant)	12-oz. pkg.	72.9
With chicken (Chun King)	10-oz. pkg.	70.8
With meat (Chun King)	10-oz. pkg.	63.8
With shrimp (Temple)	1 cup	51.0
Seasoning mix (Durkee)	1-oz. pkg.	10.9
RICE KRISPIES (Kellogg's)	1 oz.	24.6
RICE MIX, SPANISH (Uncle Ben's) with added butter	½ cup	23.3

*Prepared as Package Directs

Food and Description	Measure or Quantity	Carbohydrates (grams)
RICE & PEAS with MUSH-ROOMS (Green Giant)	12-oz. pkg.	61.8
RICE PILAF (Green Giant)	12-oz. pkg.	75.6
RICE, PUFFED (Checker) (Sunland) (Whiffs)	1 oz.	28.8
RICE PUDDING (Hunt's)	5-oz. can	32.0
RICE, SPANISH:		
(Heinz)	8¾-oz. can	35.6
Frozen (Green Giant)	12-oz. pkg.	57.9
Seasoning mix (Lawry's)	1½-oz. pkg.	20.7
RICE VERDI (Green Giant)	12-oz. pkg.	78.0
RIESLING WINE (Wilm) 11-14% alcohol	3 fl. oz.	3.6
RING DINGS (Drake's)	2¾-oz. cake	47.3
RIPPLE WINE, red (Gallo)	3 fl. oz.	3.4
ROAST 'n BOAST (General Foods):		
For beef	1½-oz. pkg.	26.0
For chicken	1⅜-oz. pkg.	19.3
For pork	1¾-oz. pkg.	27.3
For stew	1½-oz. pkg.	22.6
ROCKFISH, raw, meat only	any quantity	0.
ROE, cod or shad	4 oz.	1.7
ROLAIDS (Warner-Lambert)	1 piece	1.4
ROLL & BUN:		
Barbeque (Arnold)	1 bun	22.6
Brown & serve (Wonder)	1 roll	13.9
Butter crescent (Pepperidge Farm)	1 roll	15.1
Butterfly (Pepperidge Farm)	1 roll	8.4
Cinnamon nut (Pepperidge Farm)	1 bun	12.1
Club (Pepperidge Farm)	1 roll	22.5
Deli Twist (Arnold)	1 roll	17.4

*Prepared as Package Directs

Food and Description	Measure or Quantity	Carbohydrates (grams)
Diet Size (Arnold)	1 roll	6.2
Dinner (Arnold)	1 roll	10.5
Dinner (Pepperidge Farm)	1 roll	9.9
Dutch Egg, sandwich (Arnold)	1 bun	22.4
Finger:		
(Arnold) handipan	1 roll	9.6
Egg (Arnold) family	1 roll	9.5
(Sara Lee)	1 oz.	12.0
Frankfurter:		
(Arnold)	1 roll	20.6
New England (Arnold)	1 roll	22.0
(Pepperidge Farm)	1 roll	20.1
(Wonder)	1 bun	21.3
French:		
Triple (Pepperidge Farm)	1 roll	50.0
Twin (Pepperidge Farm)	1 roll	72.5
Golden Twist (Pepperidge Farm)	1 roll	15.0
Hamburger:		
(Pepperidge Farm)	1 roll	19.4
(Wonder)	1 bun	21.3
Hard (Levy's)	1 roll	37.4
Hearth (Pepperidge Farm)	1 roll	11.6
Honey, frozen (Morton)	1 serving	24.8
Kaiser, brown & serve (Arnold)	1 roll	23.2
Old fashioned (Pepperidge Farm)	1 roll	4.9
Parker (Arnold) handipan	1 roll	9.8
Parkerhouse (Sara Lee)	1 oz.	12.0
Party Pan (Pepperidge Farm):		
Plain	1 roll	5.5
Poppy	1 roll	5.4
Pecan, coffee (Pepperidge Farm)	1 bun	20.5
Sandwich, soft (Arnold)	1 roll	20.4
Sesame crisp (Pepperidge Farm):		
Mid-west	1 roll	12.3
East	1 roll	12.1
Sesame seed (Sara Lee)	1 oz.	12.0
Soft (Arnold) handipan	1 roll	9.1
ROLL DOUGH, refrigerated:		
Cinnamon with icing (Pillsbury)	1 oz.	14.0
Dinner (Pillsbury):		
Buttermilk	1 oz.	11.9

*Prepared as Package Directs

Food and Description	Measure or Quantity	Carbohydrates (grams)
Crescent	1 oz.	10.8
Parkerhouse	1 oz.	12.6
Snowflake	1 oz.	11.9
ROLL MIX (Pillsbury) hot	1 oz.	19.2
ROOT BEER SOFT DRINK:		
Sweetened:		
(Canada Dry) *Rooti*	6 fl. oz.	19.0
(Clicquot Club) (Cott) (Mission)	6 fl. oz.	21.0
(Dad's)	6 fl. oz.	19.6
(Dr. Brown's) (Hoffman) (Key Food) (Nedick's) (Waldbaum)	6 fl. oz.	19.4
(Fanta)	6 fl. oz.	19.8
(Hires)	6 fl. oz.	18.8
(Kirsch)	6 fl. oz.	17.7
(Nehi)	6 fl. oz.	24.2
(Salute)	6 fl. oz.	22.8
(Shasta) draft	6 fl. oz.	21.3
(Yukon Club)	6 fl. oz.	20.1
Low caloric:		
(Canada Dry)	6 fl. oz.	<1.0
(Clicquot Club) (Cott) (Dad's) (Hoffman) (Mission) (No-Cal) (Shasta) (Yukon Club)	6 fl. oz.	<.1
ROSE WINE:		
(Antinori) 12% alcohol	3 fl. oz.	6.3
(Gallo) 13% alcohol	3 fl. oz.	1.9
(Great Western) 12% alcohol	3 fl. oz.	4.7
(Mogen David) 12% alcohol	3 fl. oz.	8.9
(Taylor) 12½% alcohol	3 fl. oz.	Tr.
RUSK (Nabisco)	1 piece	9.0
RUTABAGA, raw, without tops	1 lb.	42.4

S

Food and Description	Measure or Quantity	Carbohydrates (grams)
SABLEFISH, whole	any quantity	0.
SAINT-EMILION WINE (B & G) 12% alcohol	3 fl. oz.	.7

*Prepared as Package Directs

Food and Description	Measure or Quantity	Carbohydrates (grams)
SALAD DRESSING:		
Bennett's	1 T.	2.3
Blendaise (Marzetti)	1 T.	2.6
Bleu or blue cheese:		
(Kraft) Imperial	1 T.	.9
(Lawry's)	1 T.	.8
Caesar (Kraft)	1 T.	.8
Caesar (Lawry's)	1 T.	.5
Coleslaw (Kraft)	1 T.	3.4
French:		
(Best Foods) (Hellmann's)	1 T.	2.9
(Wish-Bone) deluxe	1 T.	2.3
(Wish-Bone) garlic	1 T.	3.5
Garlic, French (Hellmann's)	1 T.	3.3
Green Goddess:		
(Kraft)	1 T.	.7
(Wish-Bone)	1 T.	1.2
Italian:		
(Lawry's)	1 T.	.9
(Lawry's) with cheese	1 T.	4.7
(Wish-Bone)	1 T.	.7
Mayonnaise, imitation (Healthlife)	.5 oz.	.9
Miracle Whip (Kraft)	1 T.	1.8
Oil & vinegar (Kraft)	1 T.	.6
Roquefort (Marzetti)	1 T.	.7
Russian (Kraft) creamy	1 T.	2.1
(Saffola)	1 T.	2.2
Thousand Island:		
(Best Foods)	1 T.	2.8
(Lawry's)	1 T.	2.3
SALAD DRESSING, DIETETIC or LOW CALORIE:		
Bleu or blue:		
(Frenchette) chunky	1 T.	1.7
(Kraft)	1 T.	.5
(Slim-ette)	1 T.	.1
Caesar (Frenchette)	1 T.	1.6
Chef style (Kraft)	1 T.	2.6
Chef's (Tillie Lewis)	1 T.	.4
Diet Mayo 7 (Bennett's)	1 T.	2.0
French:		
(Bennett's)	1 T.	3.1

*Prepared as Package Directs

Food and Description	Measure or Quantity	Carbohydrates (grams)
(Frenchette)	1 T.	2.6
Green Goddess (Slim-ette)	1 T.	.5
Italian:		
Italianette (Frenchette)	1 T.	1.5
(Tillie Lewis)	1 T.	.3
(Wish-Bone)	1 T.	.6
Mayonette Gold (Frenchette)	1 T.	1.9
Thousand Island:		
(Frenchette)	1 T.	3.0
(Kraft)	1 T.	2.3
SALAD SEASONING (Durkee)	1 tsp.	.7
SALAMI:		
Cotto, all meat (Oscar Mayer)	.8-oz. slice	.4
Dilusso Genoa (Hormel)	1 oz.	<1.0
Machiaeh Brand, pure beef (Oscar Mayer)	.8-oz. slice	.8
SALISBURY STEAK:		
(Banquet)	2-lb. pkg.	46.5
(Holloway House)	7-oz. steak	18.9
(Swanson) *Hungry Man*	17-oz. dinner	63.1
(Morton) 3-course	1-lb. 1-oz. dinner	66.6
SALMON .w	any quantity	0.
SALMO.., SMOKED:		
Lox, drained (Vita)	4-oz. jar	.2
Nova, drained (Vita)	4-oz. can	1.0
SALT:		
Butter flavored (Durkee)	1 tsp.	<.1
Garlic (Lawry's)	2.9-oz. pkg.	22.9
Onion (Lawry's)	3-oz. pkg.	22.0
Seasoned (Lawry's)	3-oz. pkg.	2.3
SALT PORK	any quantity	0.
SANDWICH SPREAD:		
(Kraft)	1 oz.	5.6
(Nalley's)	1 oz.	7.0
Corned beef (Carnation)	7½-oz. can	18.5

*Prepared as Package Directs

Food and Description	Measure or Quantity	Carbohydrates (grams)
Ham salad (Carnation)	7½-oz. can	20.0
Tuna salad (Carnation)	7½-oz. can	21.0
SANGRIA MIX (Party Tyme)	½-oz. pkg.	13.7
SARDINE, Norwegian, canned:		
In mustard sauce (Underwood)	3¾-oz. can	2.3
In oil, drained (Underwood)	3¾-oz. can	.2
In tomato sauce (Underwood)	3¾-oz. can	4.3
SAUCE:		
A1	1 T.	3.4
Barbecue:		
(French's) smoky	1 T.	3.7
(General Foods) hickory smoke, *Open Pit*	1 T.	6.5
(Heinz) with onions, hickory smoke	1 T.	2.8
(Kraft) hickory smoke	1 T.	7.9
Escoffier Sauce Diable	1 T.	4.1
Escoffier Sauce Robert	1 T.	5.7
Famous (Durkee)	1 T.	3.3
57 (Heinz)	1 T.	2.6
H.P. Steak Sauce (Lea & Perrins)	1 T.	4.8
Marinara (Chef Boy-Ar-Dee)	15-oz. can	43.6
Seafood cocktail (Crosse & Blackwell)	1 T.	4.9
Sloppy Joe (Contadina)	1 T.	2.0
Soy (Chun King)	1 T.	.3
Steak (Crosse & Blackwell)	1 T.	4.8
Sweet & sour (La Choy)	1 T.	6.9
Tartar (Best Foods) (Hellmann's)	1 T.	.2
White, medium	1 cup	22.4
Worcestershire (Lea & Perrins)	1 T.	3.0
SAUCE MIX:		
*A la King (Durkee)	1.1-oz. pkg.	13.7
*Barbecue (Kraft)	1 oz.	7.9
Cheese (French's)	1¼-oz. pkg.	11.2
Hollandaise (French's)	1⅛-oz. pkg.	6.8
*Mushroom (Betty Crocker)	1 cup	20.0
*Sour cream (Kraft)	1 oz.	4.1

*Prepared as Package Directs

Food and Description	Measure or Quantity	Carbohydrates (grams)
Stroganoff (French's)	1¾-oz. pkg.	21.0
*Sweet-sour (Durkee)	2-oz. pkg.	44.6
*White (Durkee)	1½-oz. pkg.	25.0
SAUERKRAUT (Stokely-Van Camp)	1 cup	8.8
SAUSAGE:		
Breakfast (Hormel)	8-oz. can	.7
Brown 'n serve (Hormel)	1 piece	.2
In sauce, canned (Prince)	3.7-oz. can	4.2
SAUTERNES:		
(B & G) 13% alcohol	3 fl. oz.	7.6
(Gallo) haut, 12% alcohol	3 fl. oz.	2.0
(Taylor) 12½% alcohol	3 fl. oz.	2.9
SCALLOP:		
Raw, muscle only	1 lb.	14.8
Frozen:		
Breaded, fried (Mrs. Paul's)	7-oz. pkg.	45.5
Crisps (Gorton)	7-oz. pkg.	16.0
SCOTCH SOUR COCKTAIL:		
(National Distillers) *Duet*, 12½% alcohol	8-fl.-oz. can	25.6
(Party Tyme) 12½% alcohol	2 fl. oz.	5.7
SCRAPPLE (Oscar Mayer)	4 oz.	7.0
SCREWDRIVER:		
(National Distillers) *Duet*, 12½% alcohol	8-fl.-oz. can	25.6
(Party Tyme) 12½% alcohol	2 fl. oz.	6.4
Mix (Bar-Tender's)	1 serving	17.4
SEABASS, WHITE, raw	any quantity	0.
SEAFOOD PLATTER, fried (Mrs. Paul's)	9-oz. pkg.	57.6
SENGALESE SOUP (Crosse & Blackwell)	13-oz. can	13.6
SESAME SEED, hulled	1 oz.	5.0

*Prepared as Package Directs

Food and Description	Measure or Quantity	Carbohydrates (grams)
SEVEN-UP:		
Regular	6 fl. oz.	18.0
Low calorie	6 fl. oz.	5.1
SHAD, raw, whole	any quantity	0.
SHAKE 'N BAKE:		
Chicken-coating	2⅜-oz. pkg.	40.0
Fish-coating	2-oz. pkg.	33.0
Hamburger-coating	2-oz. pkg.	31.6
Pork-coating	2⅜-oz. pkg.	46.3
SHALLOT, raw	4 oz.	16.8
SHERBET:		
(Borden)	1 pt.	103.6
(Meadow Gold)	1 pt.	54.8
(Sealtest)	1 pt.	106.0
SHERRY:		
Cocktail (Gold Seal) 19% alcohol	3 fl. oz.	1.6
Cream:		
(Gallo) 20% alcohol	3 fl. oz.	8.3
(Great Western) Solera, 19% alcohol	3 fl. oz.	11.6
(Taylor) 19½% alcohol	3 fl. oz.	11.3
Dry:		
(Italian Swiss Colony-Gold Medal) 19.7% alcohol	3 fl. oz.	1.7
(Williams & Humbert) 20½% alcohol	3 fl. oz.	4.5
Dry Sack (Williams & Humbert) 20½% alcohol	3 fl. oz.	4.5
Medium:		
(Italian Swiss Colony-Private Label) 19.8% alcohol	3 fl. oz.	2.8
(Taylor) 19½% alcohol	3 fl. oz.	7.1
SHREDDED WHEAT:		
(Kellogg's) Mini-Wheats	1 oz.	23.6
(Nabisco)	1 biscuit	18.7
(Nabisco) Spoon Size	1 oz.	22.6
(Quaker)	2 biscuits	28.7

*Prepared as Package Directs

Food and Description	Measure or Quantity	Carbohydrates (grams)
SHRIMP:		
Raw, whole	1 lb.	4.7
Cocktail, tiny, drained (Icy Point) (Pillar Rock) (Snow Mist)	4½-oz. can	.8
Frozen:		
Breaded (Gorton)	1-lb. pkg.	92.0
Scampi (Gorton)	7½-oz. pkg.	14.0
SHRIMP CAKE (Mrs. Paul's)	10-oz. pkg.	61.3
SHRIMP COCKTAIL:		
(Sau-Sea)	4-oz. jar	20.6
(Sea Snack)	4-oz. jar	14.8
SHRIMP DINNER:		
Morton)	7¾-oz. dinner	37.3
(Swanson)	8-oz. dinner	41.5
SHRIMP PASTE	1 oz.	.4
SHRIMP PUFF (Durkee)	1 piece	3.0
SLENDER (Carnation):		
Dry, chocolate	1 pkg.	15.3
Liquid, any flavor	10-fl.-oz. can	28.8
SLIM JIM	1 piece	.4
SLOPPY JOE:		
(French's)	1½-oz. pkg.	26.0
(Lawry's)	1½-oz. pkg.	27.7
SMELT, raw, whole	any quantity	0.
SMOKIE SAUSAGE:		
(Oscar Mayer):		
8 links per ¾ lb.	1 link	1.0
7 links per 5 oz.	1 link	.5
(Wilson)	1 oz.	.5
SNO BALL (Hostess)	1 cake	25.8
SOAVE WINE (Antinori) 12% alcohol	3 fl. oz.	6.3

*Prepared as Package Directs

Food and Description	Measure or Quantity	Carbohydrates (grams)
SOFT SWIRL (Jell-O):		
*All flavors except chocolate	½ cup	25.8
*Chocolate	½ cup	27.4
SOLE:		
Raw	any quantity	0.
Frozen:		
(Gorton)	1-lb. pkg.	0.
(Weight Watchers)	18-oz. dinner	18.4
In lemon butter (Gorton)	9-oz. pkg.	6.0
SOUP BASE (Wyler's) beef & chicken	1 tsp.	3.3
SOUTHERN COMFORT:		
86 proof	1 fl. oz.	3.5
100 proof	1 fl. oz.	3.5
SOYBEAN:		
Young seeds, raw	1 lb.	31.7
Mature seeds, raw	1 lb.	152.0
Roasted, *Soy Town*	1 oz.	5.1
SPAGHETTI, dry	1 oz.	21.3
SPAGHETTI DINNER:		
*With meat balls (Chef Boy-Ar-Dee)	8¾-oz. pkg.	62.0
*With meat sauce (Kraft) *Deluxe*	8 oz.	46.2
Frozen, with meat balls:		
(Banquet)	11.5-oz. dinner	57.2
(Morton)	11-oz. dinner	55.9
(Swanson)	12-oz. dinner	44.4
SPAGHETTI & FRANKFURTERS (Heinz)	8½-oz. can	28.2
SPAGHETTI & GROUND BEEF (Chef Boy-Ar-Dee)	15-oz. can	52.8
SPAGHETTI & MEATBALLS:		
Canned:		
(Austex)	15-oz. can	48.5
(Franco-American)	1 cup	24.3

*Prepared as Package Directs

Food and Description	Measure or Quantity	Carbohydrates (grams)
SpaghettiO's (Franco-American)	1 cup	23.0
Frozen (Buitoni)	8 oz.	31.2
SPAGHETTI with MEAT SAUCE:		
Canned (Heinz)	8½-oz. can	26.3
Frozen:		
(Banquet)	2-lb. pkg.	104.0
(Kraft)	12½-oz. pkg.	48.9
(Morton)	20-oz. casserole	72.2
*SPAGHETTI MIX (Kraft)	4 oz.	22.2
SPAGHETTI SAUCE:		
Clam, red (Buitoni)	4 oz.	1.4
Clam, white (Buitoni)	4 oz.	2.2
Italian (Contadina)	4 fl. oz.	12.0
Meat:		
(Chef Boy-Ar-Dee)	15-oz. can	40.4
(Prince)	1 cup	22.0
Meatball (Chef Boy-Ar-Dee)	15-oz. can	63.6
Meatless or plain (Heinz)	1 cup	30.8
Mushroom (Chef Boy-Ar-Dee)	15-oz. can	45.6
SPAGHETTI SAUCE MIX:		
Italian (French's)	1½-oz. pkg.	22.6
*Prepared with or without oil (Spatini)	1 cup	18.0
With mushrooms (Lawry's)	1½-oz. pkg.	22.6
SPAGHETTI SAUCE WITH TOMATO:		
(Van Camp)	1 cup	33.8
With cheese (Chef Boy-Ar-Dee)	40-oz. can	159.0
SPAM:		
Regular	3 oz.	3.2
Spread	1 oz.	0.
SPANISH-STYLE VEGETABLES (Birds Eye)	10-oz. pkg.	21.3
SPECIAL K (Kellogg's)	1 oz.	20.9
*SPICE CAKE MIX (Duncan Hines)	1 cake	420.0

*Prepared as Package Directs

Food and Description	Measure or Quantity	Carbohydrates (grams)
SPINACH:		
Raw, packaged	1 lb.	19.5
Canned (Stokely-Van Camp)	1 cup	6.6
Frozen:		
(Birds Eye)	10-oz. pkg.	8.1
In cream sauce (Green Giant)	10-oz. pkg.	15.0
Leaf (Birds Eye)	10-oz. pkg.	9.3
Leaf, creamed (Birds Eye)	9-oz. pkg.	16.2
Leaf, in butter sauce (Green Giant)	10-oz. pkg.	12.0
SPINACH SOUFFLE (Stouffer's)	12-oz. pkg.	29.0
SPOT, raw, fillets	any quantity	0.
SPRITE, soft drink	6 fl. oz.	18.1
SQUAB, dressed	any quantity	0.
SQUASH, SUMMER:		
Fresh, crookneck & straightneck	1 lb.	19.1
Fresh, scallop	1 lb.	22.7
Fresh, zucchini & cocozelle	1 lb.	15.5
Canned, zucchini in tomato sauce (Del Monte)	1 cup	11.2
Frozen:		
Parmesan, zucchini (Mrs. Paul's)	12-oz. pkg.	16.0
Summer squash (Birds Eye)	10-oz. pkg.	6.9
SQUASH, WINTER:		
Fresh, acorn	1 lb.	38.6
Fresh, butternut	1 lb.	44.4
Fresh, hubbard	1 lb.	28.1
Frozen (Birds Eye)	12-oz. pkg.	27.3
*START	½ cup	14.9
STRAWBERRY:		
Fresh, whole	1 lb.	36.6
Frozen:		
Whole (Birds Eye)	1-lb. pkg.	106.4
Halves (Birds Eye)	1-lb. pkg.	119.7

*Prepared as Package Directs

Food and Description	Measure or Quantity	Carbohydrates (grams)
STRAWBERRY ICE CREAM:		
(Meadow Gold) 10% fat	1 pt.	64.0
(Sealtest)	1 pt.	78.0
STRAWBERRY PIE:		
(Morton)	20-oz. pie	220.8
Cream (Morton)	14.4-oz. pie	129.6
STRAWBERRY PIE FILLING:		
(Comstock)	1 cup	79.2
(Lucky Leaf)	8 oz.	60.0
STRAWBERRY-RHUBARB PIE:		
(Morton)	46-oz. pie	486.4
(Mrs. Smith's)	10″ pie	480.0
STRAWBERRY-RHUBARB PIE FILLING (Lucky Leaf)	8 oz.	62.8
STRAWBERRY SOFT DRINK:		
Sweetened:		
(Canada Dry) (Fanta)	6 fl. oz.	22.0
(Clicquot Club) (Cott) (Mission)	6 fl. oz.	20.0
(Fanta)	6 fl. oz.	22.7
(Hoffman)	6 fl. oz.	22.3
(Shasta)	6 fl. oz.	20.3
(Yoo-Hoo)	6 fl. oz.	18.0
High-protein (Yoo-Hoo)	6 fl. oz.	24.6
(Yukon Club)	6 fl. oz.	23.0
Low calorie:		
(Canada Dry)	6 fl. oz.	<1.0
(Clicquot Club) (Cott) (Mission)	6 fl. oz.	.5
(Shasta)	6 fl. oz.	<.1
STRAWBERRY TURNOVER (Pepperidge Farm)	1 turnover	34.5
STRUDEL (Pepperidge Farm):		
Apple	1 strudel	156.0
Blueberry	1 strudel	170.4
Cherry	1 strudel	160.8
Pineapple-cheese	1 strudel	127.2
STURGEON, raw	any quantity	0.

*Prepared as Package Directs

Food and Description	Measure or Quantity	Carbohydrates (grams)
SUCCOTASH, frozen (Birds Eye)	10-oz. pkg.	58.2
SUGAR:		
Brown	1 lb.	437.3
Confectioners' or granulated	1 lb.	451.3
Maple	1 lb.	408.0
SUGAR CHEX, cereal	1 oz.	23.4
SUGAR FROSTED FLAKES (Kellogg's)	1 oz.	25.2
SUGAR JETS (General Mills)	1 oz.	23.7
SUGAR POPS (Kellogg's)	1 oz.	25.6
SUGAR SMACKS (Kellogg's)	1 oz.	25.3
SUGAR SPARKLED TWINKLES (General Mills)	1 oz.	24.2
SUGAR SUBSTITUTE:		
(Adolph's); *Sweetnin* (Tillie Lewis)	1 tsp.	0.
Superose (Whitlock); (Weight Watchers)	1 packet	.9
SUNFLOWER SEED:		
In hulls	4 oz.	12.2
Hulled	1 oz.	5.6
SWEETBREADS, raw	any quantity	0.
SWEET POTATO:		
Raw	1 lb.	96.6
Canned:		
Heavy syrup (Del Monte)	½ cup	33.7
Vacuum pack (Taylor's)	½ cup	32.0
Frozen:		
Candied (Mrs. Paul's)	12-oz. pkg.	135.0
Candied yams (Birds Eye)	12-oz. pkg.	159.9
With brown sugar glaze (Birds Eye)	10-oz. pkg.	92.1

*Prepared as Package Directs

Food and Description	Measure or Quantity	Carbohydrates (grams)
SWISS STEAK, frozen:		
(Stouffer's)	10-oz. pkg.	14.0
Dinner (Swanson)	10-oz. dinner	35.0
SWORDFISH, raw	any quantity	0.

T

Food and Description	Measure or Quantity	Carbohydrates (grams)
TABASCO	¼ tsp.	<.1
TACO, beef, frozen (Patio)	13½-oz. pkg.	90.6
TACO FILLING (Gebhardt)	4 oz.	12.0
TACO SEASONING MIX:		
(French's)	1¾-oz. pkg.	23.8
(Lawry's)	1¼-oz. pkg.	21.8
TAMALE:		
(Armour Star)	15½-oz. can	63.2
(Wilson)	15½-oz. can	63.3
Frozen (Banquet) buffet	2-lb. pkg.	138.8
***TANG,** orange	½ cup	14.7
TANGELO, juice from fruit	1 lb.	24.6
TANGERINE or MANDARIN ORANGE	1 lb.	38.9
***TANGERINE JUICE** (Minute Maid) (Snow Crop)	½ cup	13.9
TAPIOCA (Minute Tapioca)	1 T.	10.0
TAPIOCA PUDDING:		
Chilled (Sealtest)	4 oz.	21.7
Canned (Hunt's)	5-oz. can	25.6
*Mix, fluffy (Minute Tapioca)	½ cup	20.1
TEA:		
(Lipton)	1 bag	0.
Instant:		
Nestea, any flavor	1 tsp.	<.1
*Lemon flavored (Lipton)	1 cup	.9

*Prepared as Package Directs

Food and Description	Measure or Quantity	Carbohydrates (grams)
TEAM	1 oz.	24.2
TEA MIX, iced:		
Nestea	3 tsp.	15.1
*Lemon flavored (Lipton)	1 cup	25.5
THICK & FROSTY (General Foods)	1 cup	37.7
THUNDERBIRD WINE (Gallo):		
14% alcohol	3 fl. oz.	8.1
20% alcohol	3 fl. oz.	7.5
THURINGER, sausage, all meat (Oscar Mayer)	.8-oz. slice	.3
TIA MARIA (Hiram Walker)		
63 proof	1 fl. oz.	10.0
TILEFISH, raw	any quantity	0.
TOASTER CAKE:		
Corn Treats (Arnold)	1.1-oz. piece	17.1
Toastee (Howard Johnson's):		
Blueberry	1 piece	17.0
Cinnamon raisin	1 piece	17.3
Corn	1 piece	18.2
Orange	1 piece	15.5
Pound	1 piece	15.9
Toastette (Nabisco):		
Apple	1 piece	32.3
Blueberry	1 piece	33.0
Brown sugar, cinnamon	1 piece	31.9
Cherry	1 piece	32.7
Orange marmalade	1 piece	32.1
Peach, strawberry	1 piece	32.7
Toast-r-Cake (Thomas):		
Bran	1 piece	19.6
Corn	1 piece	18.1
Orange	1 piece	17.9
TOASTERINO, frozen (Buitoni):		
Cheese, grilled	4 oz.	37.9
Pizzaburger	4 oz.	29.8
Sloppy Joe	4 oz.	33.8

*Prepared as Package Directs

Food and Description	Measure or Quantity	Carbohydrates (grams)
TOMATO:		
Fresh, green	1 lb.	21.1
Fresh, ripe	1 lb.	21.3
Canned:		
Sliced (Contadina)	1 cup	16.8
Stewed (Del Monte)	1 cup	13.6
Whole (Stokely-Van Camp)	1 cup	9.8
TOMATO JUICE:		
(Heinz)	5½-fl.-oz. can	6.6
(Hunt's)	5½-fl.-oz. can	7.2
TOMATO JUICE COCKTAIL, *Snap-E-Tom*	6 fl. oz.	9.3
TOMATO PASTE (Contadina)	6-oz. can	29.4
TOMATO PUREE (Contadina)	1 cup	20.0
TOMATO SALAD, jellied (Contadina)	1 cup	27.2
TOMATO SAUCE:		
(Contadina)	1 cup	16.8
(Del Monte) plain	1 cup	12.7
(Del Monte) mushrooms	1 cup	17.0
(Del Monte) onions	1 cup	18.5
(Del Monte) with tomato tidbits	1 cup	21.8
(Hunt's) plain	1 cup	18.7
(Hunt's) herb	1 cup	27.0
(Hunt's) special	1 cup	27.2
(Hunt's) with bits	1 cup	19.4
(Hunt's) with cheese	1 cup	20.6
(Hunt's) with mushrooms	1 cup	19.8
(Hunt's) with onions	1 cup	24.5
TOMATO SOUP:		
(Campbell)	1 can	28.0
(Heinz) *Great American*	1 cup	26.3
Bisque (Campbell)	1 can	41.8
TOMATO SOUP MIX:		
(Lipton) *Cup-a-Soup*	1 pkg.	17.3
*Vegetable, with noodles (Lipton)	1 cup	11.7

*Prepared as Package Directs

Food and Description	Measure or Quantity	Carbohydrates (grams)
TOM COLLINS MIX (Party Tyme)	½-oz. pkg.	13.3
TOM COLLINS (Canada Dry)	6 fl. oz.	15.0
TONGUE, raw:		
Beef	1 lb.	1.4
Calf	1 lb.	3.1
Lamb	1 lb.	1.7
TONGUE, CANNED (Hormel)	12-oz. can	.7
TOPPING:		
Butterscotch (Kraft)	1 oz.	18.9
Caramel (Kraft)	1 oz.	18.7
Chocolate fudge (Hershey's)	1 oz.	15.8
Marshmallow creme (Kraft)	1 oz.	22.9
Pecan in syrup (Smucker's)	1 T.	8.9
Pineapple (Kraft)	1 oz.	19.7
Walnut (Kraft)	1 oz.	14.3
TOPPING, WHIPPED:		
(Birds Eye) *Cool Whip*	1 T.	1.1
(Lucky Whip)	1 T.	.5
TOPPING, WHIPPED, MIX:		
*(Dream Whip)	1 T.	1.2
*(Lucky Whip)	1 T.	1.0
TOTAL (General Mills)	1 oz.	23.0
TRIPE, beef, raw	any quantity	0.
TRIPLE SEC LIQUEUR:		
(Bols) 78 proof	1 fl. oz.	8.8
(Garnier) 60 proof	1 fl. oz.	8.5
(Hiram Walker) 80 proof	1 fl. oz.	9.8
TRIX (General Mills)	1 oz.	25.2
TROUT:		
Raw, brook, whole	1 lb.	0.
Frozen, boned	5-oz. trout	2.7
TUNA, raw	any quantity	0.

*Prepared as Package Directs

Food and Description	Measure or Quantity	Carbohydrates (grams)
TUNA CAKE (Mrs. Paul's)	10-oz. pkg.	47.1
TUNA PIE:		
(Banquet)	8-oz. pie	40.2
(Morton)	8-oz. pie	35.8
TURBOT, GREENLAND:		
Raw, whole	1 lb.	0.
(Weight Watchers)	18-oz. dinner	17.4
With apple (Weight Watchers)	9½-oz. luncheon	11.0
TURKEY, raw	any quantity	0.
TURKEY DINNER, frozen:		
(Banquet)	11.5-oz. dinner	28.2
(Morton) 3-course	1-lb. 1-oz. dinner	79.4
(Swanson) 3-course	16-oz. dinner	54.5
(Weight Watchers)	18-oz. dinner	12.4
TURKEY FRICASSEE (Lynden Farms)	14.5-oz. can	28.8
TURKEY PIE, frozen:		
(Banquet)	2-lb. 4-oz. pie	135.2
(Swanson) deep-dish	1-lb. pie	63.8
TURKEY TETRAZZINI (Stouffer's)	12-oz. pkg.	68.7
TURNIP, raw, without tops	1 lb.	25.7
TURNIP GREENS, leaves & stems:		
Fresh	1 lb.	19.0
Frozen, chopped (Birds Eye)	10-oz. pkg.	8.1
TURTLE, GREEN, in shell	any quantity	0.
TWINKIE (Hostess) 12 to pkg.	1 cake	22.1

V

VALPOLICELLA WINE (Antinori)	3 fl. oz.	6.3
VANDERMINT (Park Avenue Imports) 60 proof	1 fl. oz.	10.2

*Prepared as Package Directs

Food and Description	Measure or Quantity	Carbohydrates (grams)
VANILLA ICE CREAM:		
(Borden) 10.5% fat	1 pt.	63.2
French (Prestige)	1 pt.	63.2
Fudge royale (Sealtest)	1 pt.	72.8
VANILLA ICE MILK (Borden)		
Lite-line	1 pt.	68.8
VANILLA PUDDING:		
Canned (Del Monte)	5-oz. can	32.8
Canned (Hunt's)	5-oz. can	30.2
Canned (My-T-Fine)	5-oz. can	34.4
VANILLA PUDDING or PIE FILLING MIX (Royal)	½ cup	27.5
VEAL, raw	any quantity	0.
VEAL DINNER:		
Parmigiana (Swanson)	12¼-oz. dinner	47.7
Breaded veal with spaghetti in tomato sauce (Swanson)	8¼-oz. pkg.	24.9
V-8 (Campbell)	¾ cup	6.0
VEGETABLES, MIXED:		
(Veg-All)	½ cup	7.8
Chinese, Chop Suey (Hung's)	4 oz.	3.0
Frozen:		
(Birds Eye)	10-oz. pkg.	37.2
In butter sauce (Green Giant)	10-oz. pkg.	27.6
Jubilee (Birds Eye)	10-oz. pkg.	56.7
VEGETABLE SOUP:		
Canned, regular pack:		
*(Campbell) old fashioned	1 cup	8.9
*Beef (Heinz)	1 cup	9.6
With beef broth (Heinz) *Great American*	1 cup	18.4
Vegetarian:		
*(Campbell)	1 cup	11.8
*(Heinz)	1 cup	14.2
*Canned, dietetic pack (Slim-ette)	8 oz.	9.9

*Prepared as Package Directs

Food and Description	Measure or Quantity	Carbohydrates (grams)
VENISON, raw	any quantity	0.
VERMOUTH:		
Dry & extra dry:		
(C & P) 19% alcohol	3 fl. oz.	3.0
(Lejon) 18.5% alcohol	3 fl. oz.	2.2
(Noilly Pratt) 19% alcohol	3 fl. oz.	1.6
Sweet:		
(C & P) 16% alcohol	3 fl. oz.	14.4
(Lejon) 18.5% alcohol	3 fl. oz.	11.4
(Noilly Pratt) 16% alcohol	3 fl. oz.	12.1
VERNORS, soft drink:		
Regular	6 fl. oz.	16.8
Low calorie	6 fl. oz.	<.1
VICHYSSOISE SOUP (Crosse & Blackwell)	13-oz. can	18.8
VIENNA SAUSAGE:		
(Armour Star)	5-oz. can	0.
(Van Camp)	1 oz.	<.1
VINEGAR:		
Cider	½ cup	7.1
Distilled	½ cup	6.0
VODKA SCREWDRIVER (Old Mr. Boston) 25 proof	3 fl. oz.	10.5

W

WAFFLE, frozen, original (Aunt Jemima)	2 sections	16.2
WALNUT, English or Persian:		
In shell	1 lb.	32.2
Shelled	½ lb.	35.8
(Diamond)	3-oz. bag	15.0
WATER CHESTNUT, CHINESE, raw	1 lb.	66.4
WATERCRESS, raw	½ lb.	6.2

*Prepared as Package Directs

Food and Description	Measure or Quantity	Carbohydrates (grams)
WATERMELON, whole	1 lb.	13.4
WATERMELON RIND (Crosse & Blackwell)	1 T.	9.3
WELSH RAREBIT, canned (Snow)	4 oz.	8.4
WHEATENA	½ cup	18.1
WHEAT GERM, cereal (Kretschmer)	1 oz.	12.6
WHEATIES (General Mills)	1 oz.	23.1
WHEAT, PUFFED, cereal (Quaker)	1 oz.	22.4
WHIP 'N CHILL (Jell-O):		
All flavors except chocolate	½ cup (3 oz.)	19.3
Chocolate	½ cup (3 oz.)	22.0
WHISKEY SOUR:		
(Hiram Walker)	3 fl. oz.	13.0
(National Distillers) *Duet,*		
12½% alcohol	8-fl.-oz. can	17.6
Mix (Bar-Tender's)	1 serving	17.2
Mix (Party Tyme)	½-oz. pkg.	13.5
WHITEFISH, LAKE, raw	any quantity	0.
WILD RICE, raw	½ cup	61.7
WON TON SOUP, canned (Mow Sang)	10-oz. can	21.0

Y

YAM, raw, whole	1 lb.	90.5
YEAST:		
Compressed (Fleischmann's)	³/₅-oz. cake	1.9
Dry (Fleischmann's)	¼ oz.	2.9

*Prepared as Package Directs

Food and Description	Measure or Quantity	Carbohydrates (grams)
YOGURT:		
Plain:		
(Borden) Swiss style	8-oz. container	15.9
(Breakstone)	8-oz. container	12.7
(Dannon)	8-oz. container	14.1
Apricot:		
(Breakstone)	8-oz. container	37.4
(Breakstone) *Swiss Parfait*	8-oz. container	42.9
(Dannon)	8-oz. container	51.1
Blueberry:		
(Breakstone)	8-oz. container	46.3
(Breakstone) *Swiss Parfait*	8-oz. container	53.1
(Dannon)	8-oz. container	51.1
(Meadow Gold)	8-oz. container	54.0
(Meadow Gold) Swiss style	8-oz. container	49.0
(Sanna) *Swiss Miss*	4-oz. container	19.0
(Sealtest) *Light n' Lively*	8-oz. container	50.6
(SugarLo)	8-oz. container	14.6
Boysenberry:		
(Dannon)	8-oz. container	51.1
(Meadow Gold)	8-oz. container	54.0
Cherry:		
(Dannon)	8-oz. container	51.1
(Meadow Gold)	8-oz. container	54.0
Dark (SugarLo)	8-oz. container	14.6
Coffee (Dannon)	8-oz. container	33.3
Danny (Dannon):		
Cuplet, any flavor	4-oz. container	25.5
Frozen pop	2½-oz. pop	18.0
Lemon:		
(Breakstone) *Swiss Parfait*	8-oz. container	44.9
(Sealtest) *Light n' Lively*	8-oz. container	43.4
Mandarin orange:		
(Borden) Swiss Style	8-oz. container	45.9
(Breakstone) *Swiss Parfait*	8-oz. container	48.3
Peach:		
(Borden) Swiss style	8-oz. container	44.5
(Breakstone) *Swiss Parfait*	8-oz. container	47.4
Melba (Breakstone) *Swiss Parfait*	8-oz. container	49.4
(Meadow Gold)	8-oz. container	54.0
(Sealtest) *Light n' Lively*	8-oz. container	49.3
(SugarLo)	8-oz. container	14.6

*Prepared as Package Directs

Food and Description	Measure or Quantity	Carbohydrates (grams)
Pineapple:		
(Breakstone)	8-oz. container	37.9
(Meadow Gold)	8-oz. container	54.0
(Sealtest) *Light n' Lively*	8-oz. container	47.2
(SugarLo)	8-oz. container	14.8
Prune whip (Breakstone)	8-oz. container	41.1
Prune whip (Dannon)	8-oz. container	51.1
Raspberry:		
(Borden) Swiss style	8-oz. container	47.2
(Breakstone)	8-oz. container	45.8
Red (Breakstone) *Swiss Parfait*	8-oz. container	46.5
(Dannon)	8-oz. container	51.1
(Meadow Gold) Swiss style	8-oz. container	49.0
(Sanna) *Swiss Miss*	4-oz. container	19.0
Red (Sealtest) *Light n' Lively*	8-oz. container	41.8
(SugarLo)	8-oz. container	14.8
Strawberry:		
(Borden) Swiss style	8-oz. container	44.5
(Breakstone)	8-oz. container	43.5
(Breakstone) *Swiss Parfait*	8-oz. container	50.6
(Dannon)	8-oz. container	51.1
(Meadow Gold)	8-oz. container	54.0
(Meadow Gold) Swiss style	8-oz. container	49.0
(Sanna) *Swiss Miss*	4-oz. container	19.0
(Sealtest) *Light n' Lively*	8-oz. container	44.3
(SugarLo)	8-oz. container	13.2
Vanilla:		
(Borden) Swiss style	8-oz. container	45.4
(Breakstone)	8-oz. container	29.5
(Dannon)	8-oz. container	33.3

Z

ZWEIBACK (Nabisco)   1 piece   5.4

*Prepared as Package Directs